KEY ANATOMY FOR RADIOLOGY

KEY ANATOMY FOR RADIOLOGY

Simon Westacott MB BS, MRCP(UK)

Registrar in Radiodiagnosis
Plymouth General Hospital
Plymouth

John R. W. Hall MB BS, MRCP(UK)

Registrar in Radiodiagnosis
Plymouth General Hospital
Plymouth

HEINEMANN PROFESSIONAL PUBLISHING

Heinemann Medical Books
An imprint of Heinemann Professional Publishing Ltd
Halley Court, Jordan Hill, Oxford OX2 8EJ

OXFORD   LONDON   MELBOURNE   AUCKLAND

First published 1988

British Library Cataloguing in Publication Data
Westacott, Simon
  Key anatomy for radiology.
  1. Man. Anatomy
  I. Title   II. Hall, John R. W.
  611

ISBN 0 433 00043 0

Typeset by Tecset Limited, Wallington, Surrey
Printed in Great Britain by LR Printing Services Ltd, Crawley,
West Sussex, RH10 2QN

CONTENTS

FOREWORD

Standard textbooks of anatomy are for the most part comprehensive in their coverage, embracing the anatomy of bones, muscles and nerves in as much detail as the rest of the body. Furthermore, many are illustrated by dissection specimens. While this approach is useful to the medical student and surgeon it is less useful to the radiologist. The part 1 examination for the Fellowship of the Royal College of Radiologists requires a detailed knowledge of those aspects of anatomy which are relevant to the practice of radiology. The authors, having fairly recently passes this examination, indentified the need for a concise and relevant anatomy text. The book which has resulted testifies to their immense energy and hard work, describing as it does the salient features of modern radiological anatomy. While the authors have drawn from the experience and advice of their colleagues and teachers in the Department of Radiology in Plymouth, the book retains a fresh approach which is due entirely to their enthusiasm. The result of their work will be judged by others – perhaps most importantly by other trainees in radiology. I feel sure that they will not be disappointed.

D. E. Beckly FRCP, FRCR
Chairman
Division of Radiology
Plymouth General Hospital

PREFACE

During our radiological training we have identified the need for a textbook which gives a concise account of anatomy relevant to the practice of radiology. Although medical training provides a grounding in anatomy, the complexities of radiographic imaging and, in particular, cross-sectional imaging require a slightly different perception of the structures of the body and their relations. This book, therefore, relies heavily upon diagrams, many of which are derived directly from radiographs and scans produced in our department. Because living subjects have been used, there are a few minor differences compared to standard anatomy textbooks, particularly with respect to the vertebral levels quoted for some structures.

Each chapter and section conforms to a specific arrangement: a brief account of a structure is followed by its relations and vascular anatomy, both of which are simply listed so that they may be easily referred to (or ignored!) if required. Each structure also has a list of methods of imaging. At the time of writing, the place of magnetic resonance imaging has not been fully evaluated but, in general, wherever computed tomography is mentioned this can be taken to include magnetic resonance imaging.

Each diagram has a separate key for clarity and for the purpose of self-assessment. To avoid repetition not all the cross-sections are fully labelled, and referral to an earlier diagram may sometimes be necessary. The diagrams should be regarded as typical examples; we have made no attempt to include anatomical variants.

This book is aimed primarily at candidates for the part 1 examination for Fellowship of the Royal College of Radiologists, or equivalent, and we assume a knowledge of the fundamentals of anatomy. Nonetheless, we hope that it will be useful for other clinicians, medical students and radiographers, and that it will be a handy source of reference for practising radiologists.

Simon Westacott, John R. W. Hall, 1988

ACKNOWLEDGEMENTS

We gratefully acknowledge the help and encouragement of our colleagues and consultants at Plymouth General Hospital, particularly Dr Paul Dubbins and Dr Ross Paxton for editorial advice. We owe a special debt of gratitude to Sally Hawke for processing our words.

1 | The Thorax

The thorax consists of a bell-shaped musculoskeletal cage between the neck and the abdomen. It is divided into right and left pleural cavities, separated by the mediastinum. Each pleural cavity is limited superiorly by a suprapleural membrane attached to the transverse process of C7 and the inner border of the first rib. The mediastinum is a midline potential space between the pleural cavities and is continuous with the neck. It is bounded by the manubrium and sternum anteriorly, the vertebral column posteriorly, the diaphragm inferiorly and by parietal pleura laterally. It is divided into superior and inferior parts by a line passing between the manubriosternal junction and the lower border of T4. The inferior mediastinum is divided into anterior, middle and posterior parts.

THE LUNGS, HILA AND PLEURAE

The lungs are the organs of respiration. Each lies within its pleural cavity, lateral to the mediastinum. Each has a conical shape with an apex superiorly, a base inferiorly, a convex costal surface and a concave medial surface which is more pronounced on the left owing to the cardiac indentation.

The lung is connected to the mediastinum by the hilum on its medial surface (Figs. 1.1, 1.2). This is traversed by pulmonary arteries and veins, bronchial arteries, lymph vessels and bronchi. The hilum contains lymph nodes and connective tissue.

Each lung lies within a double layer of pleura, a serous membrane which forms a parietal lining to the pleural cavity and a visceral covering to the lung. The parietal pleura forms a reflection around the hilar vessels and extends, as an inferior fold, to form the pulmonary ligament.

The lungs are divided into lobes by fissures which are invaginations of visceral pleura into the lung substance: the left lung is divided into upper and lower lobes by an oblique fissure; the right is divided into upper, middle and lower lobes by oblique and horizontal fissures (Fig. 1.3). The lobes are subdivided into bronchopulmonary segments, each of which is a functionally independent volume of lung tissue supplied by a single segmental bronchus (Fig. 1.4) and separated from adjacent segments by connective tissue septa. Each bronchopulmonary segment is made up of several pulmonary lobules, which are the smallest functional units of the lung, corresponding to individual bronchioles.

Medial relations of the right lung (Fig. 1.5):

>   trachea
>   oesophagus
>   thymus
>   ascending aorta
>   brachiocephalic veins
>   superior vena cava
>   azygos vein
>   right atrium
>   inferior vena cava
>   intercostal vessels and nerves
>   right vagus nerve
>   right phrenic nerve
>   T1 nerve root
>   sympathetic chain
>   vertebral column

Medial relations of the left lung (Fig. 1.6):

>   oesophagus
>   thymus
>   left subclavian artery
>   left brachiocephalic vein
>   aorta
>   pulmonary trunk
>   left ventricle
>   accessory hemiazygos vein
>   thoracic duct
>   intercostal vessels and nerves
>   left vagus nerve
>   left phrenic nerve
>   T1 nerve root
>   sympathetic chain
>   vertebral column

Vascular anatomy of the lungs:

arterial: pulmonary artery
bronchial arteries, arising from the descending aorta and intercostal arteries

venous: pulmonary veins
bronchial veins, draining into the azygos and accessory hemiazygos veins

lymph: pulmonary nodes
bronchopulmonary nodes
tracheobronchial nodes
paratracheal nodes

Methods of imaging the lungs:

radiographic: plain films with standard or increased penetration or high kV
tomography
computed tomography
pulmonary arteriography
bronchography

radionuclide: ^{99m}Tc-albumin perfusion scintigraphy
^{81m}Kr ventilation scintigraphy
^{133}Xe ventilation scintigraphy
^{99m}Tc-DTPA aerosol ventilation scintigraphy

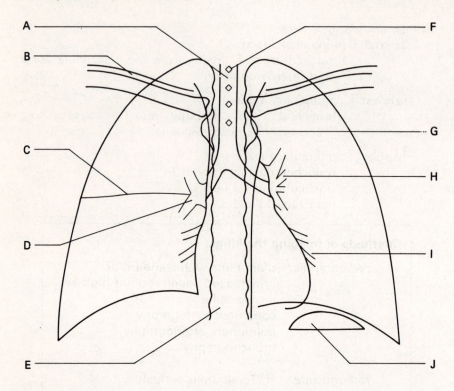

Fig. 1.1 *Frontal view of the chest*

A: trachea
B: companion shadow of the
      clavicle
C: horizontal fissure
D: right hilum
E: vertebral column

F: spinous process
G: manubrium
H: left hilum
I: inferior pulmonary vein
J: gastric air bubble

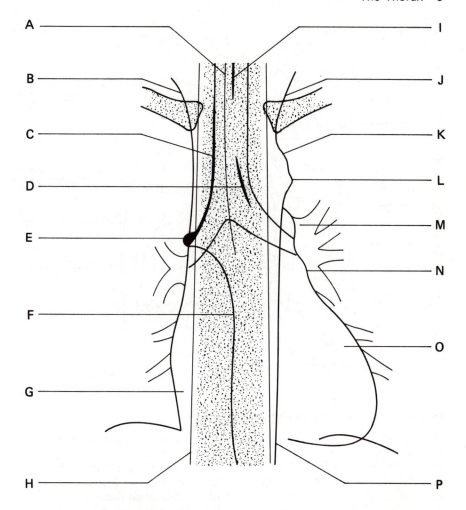

Fig. 1.2 *Frontal view of the mediastinum*

A: pleuro-oesophageal line
B: right brachiocephalic
       vein/superior vena cava
C: right tracheal stripe
D: anterior junction line
E: azygos vein
F: azygo-oesophageal line
G: right atrium
H: right paraspinal line

I: posterior junction line
J: subclavian artery
K: aortic arch
L: left superior intercostal
       vein
M: pulmonary trunk
N: left auricle
O: left ventricle
P: descending aorta

Uploaded/DISCS

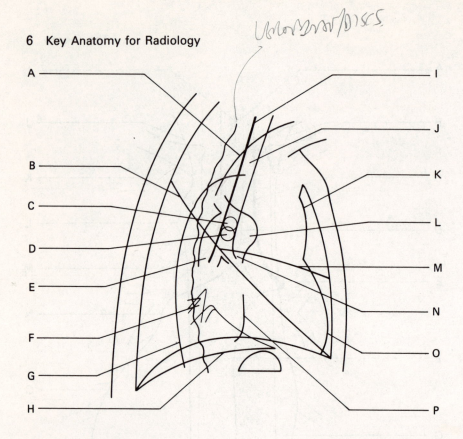

Fig. 1.3 *Lateral view of the chest*

A: axillary skin fold
B: oblique fissure
C: right upper lobe bronchus
D: left upper lobe bronchus
E: left pulmonary artery
F: inferior pulmonary veins
G: descending aorta
H: left hemidiaphragm

I: posterior tracheal stripe
J: trachea
K: ascending aorta
L: pulmonary trunk
M: horizontal fissure
N: right pulmonary artery
O: right ventricle
P: inferior vena cava

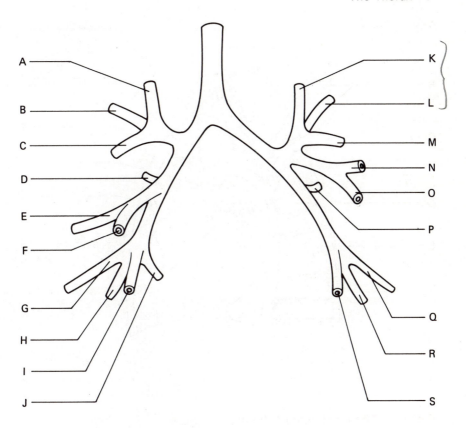

Fig. 1.4 *The segmental bronchi*

A: upper lobe, apical
B: upper lobe, posterior
C: upper lobe, anterior
D: lower lobe, apical
E: middle lobe, lateral
F: middle lobe, medial
G: lower lobe, lateral
H: lower lobe, posterior
I: lower lobe, anterior
J: lower lobe, medial

K: upper lobe, apical
L: upper lobe, posterior
M: upper lobe, anterior
N: upper lobe, superior
       lingular
O: upper lobe, inferior
       lingular
P: lower lobe, apical
Q: lower lobe, lateral
R: lower lobe, posterior
S: lower lobe, anterior

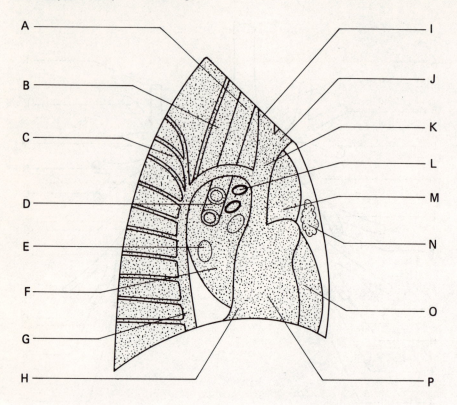

Fig. 1.5   *The right side of the mediastinum*

A:	trachea	I:	right brachiocephalic vein
B:	oesophagus	J:	left brachiocephalic vein
C:	vertebral column	K:	superior vena cava
D:	bronchi	L:	pulmonary arteries
E:	inferior pulmonary vein	M:	ascending aorta
F:	left atrium	N:	thymus
G:	azygos vein	O:	right ventricle
H:	inferior vena cava	P:	right atrium

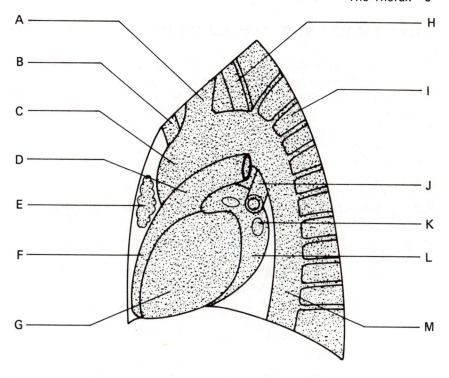

Fig. 1.6 *The left side of the mediastinum*

A: subclavian artery
B: brachiocephalic vein
C: aortic arch
D: pulmonary trunk
E: thymus
F: right ventricle
G: left ventricle

H: oesophagus
I: vertebral column
J: bronchus
K: inferior pulmonary vein
L: left atrium
M: descending aorta

THE TRACHEA AND MAIN BRONCHI

The trachea and bronchi are respiratory passages which convey air from the larynx to the alveoli of the lungs. The trachea is a tubular structure, flattened posteriorly. It lies in the midline of the neck and superior mediastinum, extending from the level of C6 to the lower border of T5, where it divides into the right and left main bronchi. Its total length is 10 cm. The main bronchi traverse the middle mediastinum and the hila to form a branching network within the lungs. The right main bronchus is 3 cm long; the left is more horizontal and is 5 cm long.

tory epithelium and reinforced, outside the lungs, by incomplete rings of elastic cartilage.

Relations of the trachea in the superior mediastinum (Figs. 1.7–1.9):

anterior:	manubrium
	right brachiocephalic vein
	superior vena cava
	brachiocephalic artery
	aortic arch
	lymph nodes
	thymus
posterior:	oesophagus
right:	azygos vein *as it curves forward to join SVC*
	right vagus nerve
	lymph nodes
	right lung
left:	left common carotid artery
	left subclavian artery
	aortic arch
	left recurrent laryngeal nerve
	lymph nodes

The main bronchi (Fig. 1.10) are related to the pulmonary vessels, most of which lie anteriorly and inferiorly. The left pulmonary artery, initially anterior, loops backward over the left main bronchus as the latter traverses the hilum. The aortic arch and descending aorta are superior and posterior relations, respectively, of the left main bronchus and the oesophagus deviates from the midline to lie behind it. The azygos vein loops forward over the right main bronchus before entering the superior vena cava.

Vascular anatomy of the trachea and proximal main bronchi:

    arterial: inferior thyroid arteries
                 bronchial arteries

    venous: inferior thyroid veins

    lymph: pretracheal nodes
                 paratracheal nodes

Methods of imaging the trachea and main bronchi:

    radiographic: plain films and tomography
                        computed tomography
                        bronchography

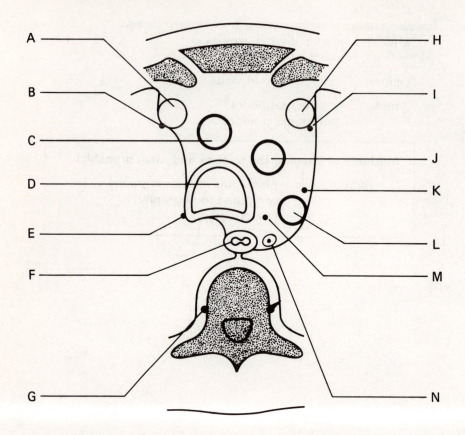

Fig. 1.7 *Cross section through the mediastinum at the level of T3*

A: right brachiocephalic vein
B: right phrenic nerve
C: brachiocephalic artery
D: trachea
E: right vagus nerve
F: oesophagus
G: right sympathetic trunk

H: left brachiocephalic vein
I: left phrenic nerve
J: left common carotid
    artery
K: left vagus nerve
L: left subclavian artery
M: left recurrent laryngeal
    nerve
N: thoracic duct

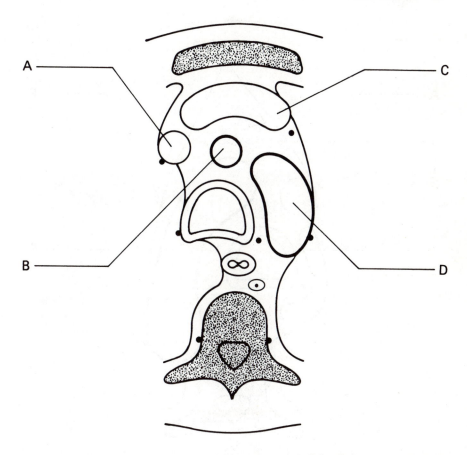

Fig. 1.8 *Cross section through the mediastinum at the level of T4*

A: right brachiocephalic vein   C: left brachiocephalic vein
B: brachiocephalic artery   D: aortic arch

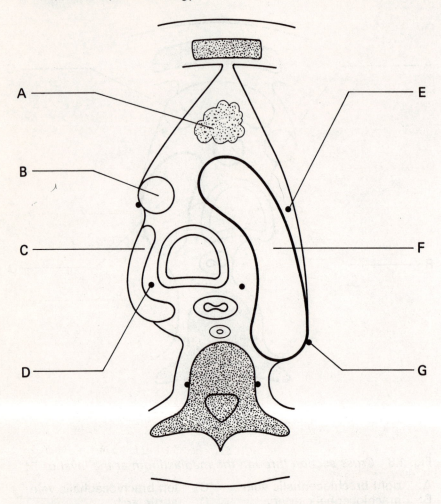

Fig. 1.9 *Cross section through the mediastinum at the level of T5*

A: thymus
B: superior vena cava
C: azygos vein
D: right vagus nerve

E: left phrenic nerve
F: aortic arch
G: left vagus nerve

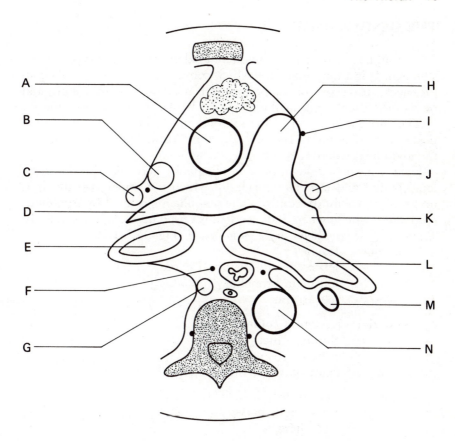

Fig. 1.10 *Cross section through the mediastinum at the level of T6*

A: ascending aorta
B: superior vena cava
C: right superior pulmonary
    vein
D: right pulmonary artery
E: right main bronchus
F: right vagus nerve
G: azygos vein

H: pulmonary trunk
I: left phrenic nerve
J: left superior pulmonary
    vein
K: left pulmonary artery
L: left main bronchus
M: left pulmonary artery
N: descending aorta

THE OESOPHAGUS

The oesophagus transmits ingested food from the pharynx to the stomach. It is a muscular tube which commences at the level of C6 in the neck, traverses the superior and posterior mediastinum and pierces the diaphragm at the level of T10. In the neck and superior mediastinum it lies close to the midline but deviates to the left in the posterior mediastinum. Its total length is 25 cm. The distal 3 cm is in the abdomen, where it is retroperitoneal.

Food is propelled down the oesophagus by peristalsis produced by longitudinal and circular muscle, of which the upper two thirds is under some voluntary control. The oesophagus is lined by squamous epithelium which, when undistended, is raised into longitudinal folds.

Relations of the oesophagus in the mediastinum (Figs. 1.7–1.10):

anterior:	trachea
	left recurrent laryngeal nerve
	left main bronchus
	left atrium
posterior:	vertebral column
	thoracic duct
	hemiazygos veins
	right posterior intercostal arteries
right:	azygos vein
	right vagus nerve
	right lung
left:	left subclavian artery
	left common carotid artery
	aortic arch
	descending aorta
	thoracic duct
	left vagus nerve
	left lung

Vascular anatomy:

arterial:	inferior thyroid arteries
	branches of the descending aorta
	bronchial arteries
	left gastric artery, arising from the coeliac axis

venous: inferior thyroid veins
            azygos vein
            hemiazygos veins
            left gastric vein, draining into the portal vein

lymph: deep cervical nodes
            posterior mediastinal nodes
            coeliac nodes

Methods of imaging the oesophagus:

radiographic: plain films and tomography
                  barium swallow
                  computed tomography

radionuclide: ^{99m}Tc-labelled colloid milk reflux
                  studies

THE THORACIC DUCT

The thoracic duct drains lymph to the venous system from the whole body with the exception of the right side of the thorax, neck and head. It commences as the continuation of the cisterna chyli, a thin-walled sac in the upper abdomen between the aorta and the right crus of the diaphragm. The duct pierces the diaphragm at the level of T12, with the aorta. It ascends in the posterior mediastinum behind the oesophagus and between the aorta and the azygos vein (Figs. 1.7–1.10, 1.17–1.20). It crosses to the left at the level of T5, then arches anteriorly and to the left in the superior mediastinum and the neck before opening into the origin of the left brachiocephalic vein at the level of C7. The duct is 45 cm long; the cisterna chyli is 6 cm long.

The remainder of the body is drained by the right lymph duct which opens into the origin of the right brachiocephalic vein.

Methods of imaging the thoracic duct:

radiographic: computed tomography
                  lymphography

THE THYMUS

The thymus is a lymphoid organ which lies predominantly in the mediastinum behind the sternum but with a variable position. It consists of two irregularly-shaped lobes connected across the midline (Figs. 1.5, 1.6, 1.9, 1.10).

The thymus consists of lymphoid and epithelial cells supported by fibrous trabeculae and contained within a fibrous capsule. In adult life the lymphoid and epithelial cells are replaced by fatty tissue.

Relations:

anterior:	lungs
	thoracic wall
posterior:	pericardium
	ascending aorta
	brachiocephalic artery
	left common carotid artery
	left brachiocephalic vein
	trachea
lateral:	lungs

Vascular anatomy:

arterial:	inferior thyroid arteries
	internal thoracic arteries
venous:	inferior thyroid veins
	internal thoracic veins
lymph:	brachiocephalic nodes
	tracheobronchial nodes
	parasternal nodes

Methods of imaging the thymus:

radiographic: plain films and tomography
computed tomography

THE HEART

The heart consists of two atria and two ventricles, chambers with muscular walls which pump blood in the systemic and pulmonary circuits. It occupies most of the middle mediastinum. It is egg-shaped, having its long axis pointing forward, downward and to the left. The apex lies above the left hemidiaphragm and the base, the origin of the great vessels, lies superiorly.

The left atrium and ventricle receive pulmonary venous blood and pump it into systemic arteries. Forward flow is ensured by the presence of the mitral and aortic valves: the mitral valve (Figs. 1.11, 1.12, 1.19) lies in the left atrioventricular orifice and has two fibrous cusps, one anterior and one posterior; the aortic valve lies in the orifice of the ascending aorta and has three cusps. The corresponding valves on the right are the tricuspid and pulmonary valves, each having three cusps. The competence of the atrioventricular valves is reinforced by tendinous cords attached to the free borders of the cusps and to papillary muscles which arise from the ventricular walls. The atria are separated by a thin-walled interatrial septum and the ventricles by a thick interventricular septum which functions as an integral part of the left ventricle and bulges into the right ventricle. These septa lie at an angle to the sagittal plane so that the left atrium and ventricle are predominantly posterior and the right atrium and ventricle are predominantly anterior (Figs. 1.17–1.20).

The heart is supported in the mediastinum by the roots of the great vessels and by the pericardium, which envelops it.

The heart is a muscular organ with specialised cells for automaticity of contraction and electrical conduction. The sinoatrial node lies in the right atrium in front of the opening of the superior vena cava and the atrioventricular node lies in the interatrial septum. From the atrioventricular node bundles of conductive fibres pass down the interventricular septum toward the apex. The atrial walls are generally smooth, whereas the ventricular walls are raised into muscular ridges. The ventricular outflow tracts, however, are smooth, forming the vestibule beneath the aortic valve and the infundibulum beneath the pulmonary valve. The origin of the ascending aorta is dilated into three sinuses corresponding to the cusps of the aortic valve. The right and left coronary arteries (Figs. 1.13, 1.14) arise from the anterior and left posterior sinuses, respectively, and run on the surface of the heart.

Relations: as for the pericardium, p.26

Vascular anatomy:

arterial: left coronary artery
            right coronary artery

venous: coronary sinus $\Big\}$ draining into the right atrium
            anterior cardiac veins

lymph: brachiocephalic nodes
            tracheobronchial nodes

Methods of imaging the heart:

radiographic: plain films and tomography
                  computed tomography
                  angiocardiography
                  coronary arteriography

ultrasonographic: real-time B-mode
                      M-mode echocardiography

radionuclide: ^{201}Tl myocardial scintigraphy
                  ^{99m}Tc-labelled red cell
                  ventriculoscintigraphy by first-
                  pass or multiple-gated acquisition
                  (MUGA)

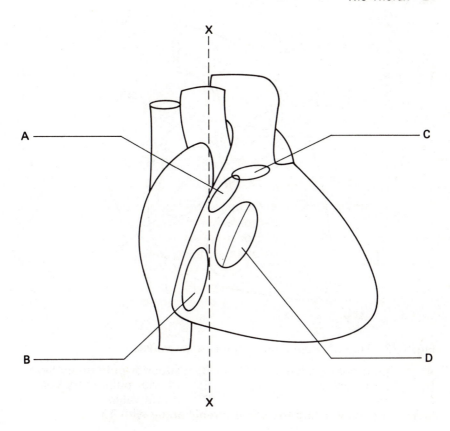

Fig. 1.11   *Frontal projection of the cardiac valves*

A: aortic valve   C: pulmonary valve
B: tricuspid valve   D: mitral valve
X–X: midline

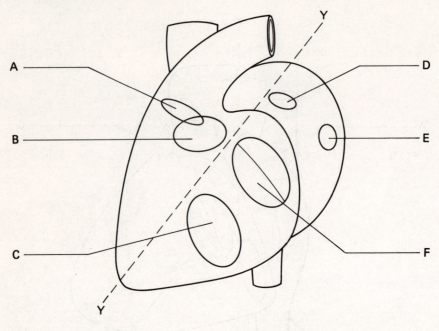

Fig. 1.12 *Lateral projection of the cardiac valves*

A: pulmonary valve   D: superior pulmonary vein
B: aortic valve   E: inferior pulmonary vein
C: tricuspid valve   F: mitral valve
Y–Y: line connecting the costophrenic angle with T5

roughly = frowe

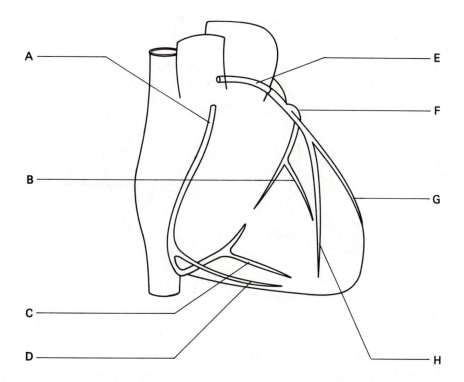

Fig. 1.13 *Frontal view of the coronary arteries*

A: right coronary artery
B: left marginal artery
C: posterior interventricular artery
D: right marginal artery

E: left coronary artery
F: circumflex artery
G: diagonal artery
H: anterior interventricular artery

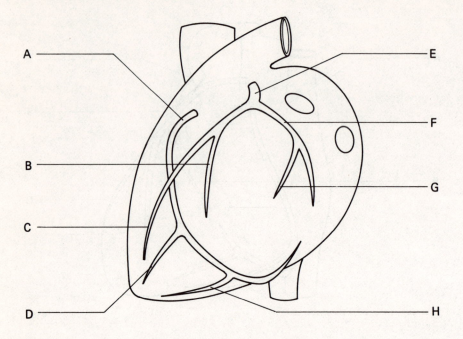

Fig. 1.14 *Lateral view of the coronary arteries*

A: right coronary artery
B: diagonal artery
C: anterior interventricular
   artery
D: right marginal artery

E: left coronary artery
F: circumflex artery
G: left marginal artery
H: posterior interventricular
   artery

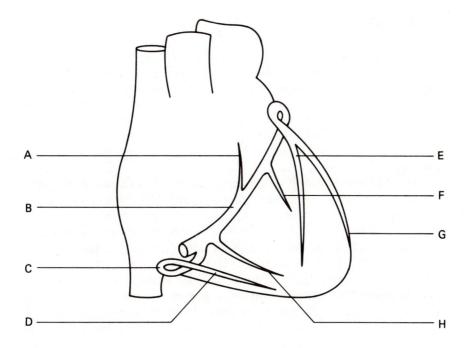

Fig. 1.15 *Frontal view of the venous drainage of the heart*

A: oblique vein
B: coronary sinus
C: small cardiac vein
D: right marginal vein

E: great cardiac vein
F: left posterior
       interventricular vein
G: left marginal vein
H: middle cardiac vein

THE PERICARDIUM

The pericardium is a sac containing the heart, coronary vessels, the roots of the aorta and pulmonary trunk, and the terminations of the venae cavae and pulmonary veins. It consists of two parts: the outer, fibrous pericardium is continuous with the fibrous adventitia of the great vessels; the inner, serous pericardium has two layers which form a parietal lining to the fibrous pericardium and the epicardium, a visceral covering to the heart. The fibrous pericardium follows the contours of the heart and extends to envelop the ends of the great vessels. The arrangement of the serous pericardium is more complex: the parietal layer forms a superior reflection which encircles the roots of the aorta and pulmonary trunk whilst the inferior reflection forms a loop around the terminations of the venae cavae and pulmonary veins (Fig. 1.16). The transverse sinus is a potential space separating the superior and inferior reflections. It is continuous with the space between the fibrous pericardium and the parietal layer of serous pericardium. The oblique sinus is a pocket-shaped potential space formed by the inferior reflection around the pulmonary veins. It is continuous with the space between the two layers of serous pericardium.

The pericardium, and therefore the heart, is supported by sterno-pericardial ligaments anteriorly, by the diaphragm inferiorly, by the roots of the aorta and pulmonary trunk superiorly and by the terminations of the venae cavae and pulmonary veins posteriorly. Elsewhere it is covered by parietal pleura.

Relations:

anterior:	thymus
	lungs
	thoracic wall
posterior:	bronchi
	oesophagus
	vagus nerves
	descending aorta
	lungs
superior:	ascending aorta
	pulmonary trunk
	superior vena cava
inferior:	inferior vena cava
	diaphragm
	liver
	stomach

lateral: musculophrenic vessels
          phrenic nerves
          lungs

Vascular anatomy:
   arterial: internal thoracic arteries
              musculophrenic arteries
              branches of the descending aorta

   venous: azygos vein
             hemiazygos veins

   lymph: brachiocephalic nodes
             posterior mediastinal nodes
             tracheobronchial nodes

Methods of imaging the pericardium:

radiographic: plain films and tomography
                 computed tomography

ultrasonographic: M-mode echocardiography

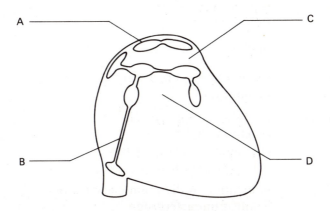

Fig. 1.16 *Reflections of the serous pericardium*

A: reflection around aorta
    and pulmonary trunk
B: reflection around
    pulmonary veins and
    venae cavae

C: transverse fissure
D: oblique sinus

THE THORACIC AORTA

The aorta conveys oxygenated blood from the left ventricle. The ascending aorta is 5 cm long and lies in the midline in the middle mediastinum. It is dilated at its origin by the three aortic sinuses corresponding to the cusps of the aortic valve and is enveloped proximally in pericardium. The aortic arch lies in the superior mediastinum. It commences behind the manubrium and arches backward and to the left, giving rise to the arteries of the neck. The descending aorta lies to the left of the midline in the posterior mediastinum and gives rise to the posterior intercostal arteries, which run in the third to eleventh intercostal spaces, the bronchial arteries and vessels supplying mediastinal structures and the diaphragm. It pierces the diaphragm at the level of T12.

Relations of the ~~aortic arch~~ (Figs. 1.6, 1.9):

ascending

anterior:	infundibulum of the right ventricle
	pulmonary trunk
	sternum
	right lung
	thymus
posterior:	left atrium
	right pulmonary artery
right:	auricle of the right atrium
	superior vena cava
	right lung
left:	pulmonary trunk

Relations of the aortic arch (Figs. 1.6, 1.9):

anterior:	manubrium
superior:	left brachiocephalic vein
	brachiocephalic artery
	left common carotid artery
	left subclavian artery
inferior:	bifurcation of the pulmonary trunk
	ligamentum arteriosum
	left recurrent laryngeal nerve
	left main bronchus

right: right lung
            superior vena cava
            trachea
            left recurrent laryngeal nerve
            oesophagus
            thoracic duct
            T4

left: left lung
            left phrenic nerve
            left vagus nerve
            left superior intercostal vein

Relations of the descending aorta in the mediastinum (Figs. 1.10, 1.17–1.20):

anterior: left pulmonary artery
            left main bronchus
            left inferior pulmonary vein
            left atrium
            oesophagus

posterior: left transverse processes

right: vertebral column
            oesophagus
            thoracic duct
            hemiazygos veins
            left sympathetic chain

left: left lung

Methods of imaging the aorta:

radiographic: plain films and tomography
                     computed tomography
                     aortography

ultrasonographic: real-time B-mode
                     Doppler

radionuclide: ^{99m}Tc-labelled red cell first-pass
                     studies

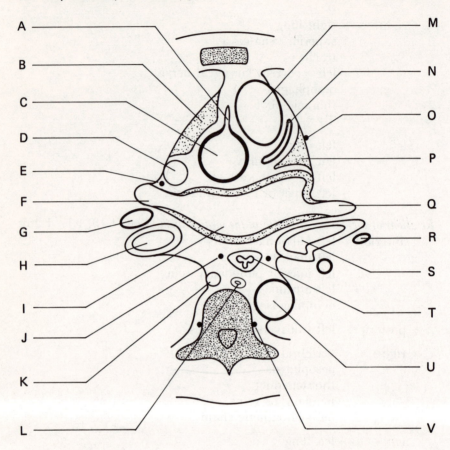

Fig. 1.17 *Cross section through the mediastinum at the level of T7*

A: right coronary artery
B: right auricle
C: ascending aorta
D: superior vena cava
E: right phrenic nerve
F: right superior pulmonary
       vein
G: right pulmonary artery
H: right main bronchus
I: left atrium
J: right vagus nerve
K: azygos vein
L: thoracic duct

M: pulmonary trunk
N: left coronary artery
O: left phrenic nerve
P: left auricle
Q: left superior pulmonary
       vein
R: left pulmonary artery
S: left main bronchus
T: oesophagus
U: descending aorta
V: left sympathetic chain

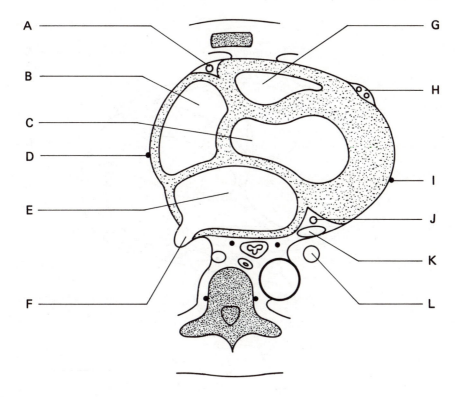

Fig. 1.18 *Cross section through the mediastinum at the level of T8*

A: right coronary artery
B: right atrium
C: vestibule of the left
    ventricle
D: right phrenic nerve
E: left atrium
F: right inferior pulmonary
    vein

G: right ventricle
H: anterior interventricular
    artery, great cardiac vein
I: left phrenic nerve
J: circumflex artery
K: coronary sinus
L: left inferior pulmonary
    vein

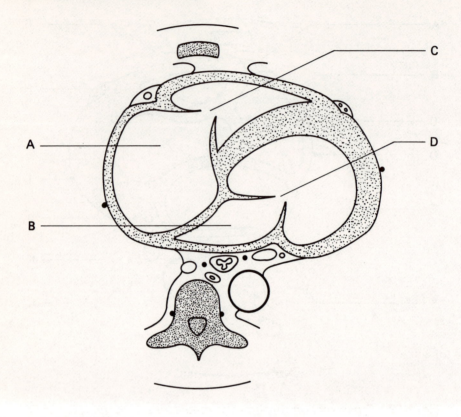

Fig 1.19 *Cross section through the mediastinum at the level of T9*

A: right atrium
B: left atrium

C: tricuspid valve
D: mitral valve

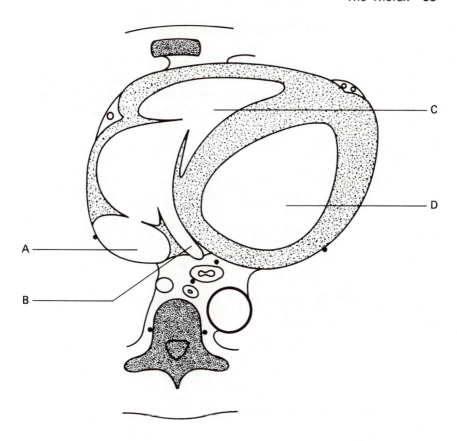

Fig. 1.20   *Cross section through the mediastinum at the level of T10*

A: inferior vena cava
B: coronary sinus

C: right ventricle
D: left ventricle

THE PULMONARY TRUNK AND ARTERIES

The pulmonary trunk conveys deoxygenated blood from the right ventricle. It is 5 cm long and enveloped in pericardium. The trunk divides into the right pulmonary artery, which runs horizontally to the right in the coronal plane, and the left pulmonary artery, which loops backward over the left main bronchus.

Relations of the pulmonary trunk (Figs. 1.10, 1.17):

anterior:	thymus
	left lung
posterior:	left coronary artery
	left atrium
right:	ascending aorta
	right coronary artery
left:	left phrenic nerve
	lung

Relations of the right pulmonary artery:

anterior:	ascending aorta
	superior vena cava
	right superior pulmonary vein
	right phrenic nerve
posterior:	right main bronchus
superior:	azygos vein
inferior:	right superior pulmonary vein

Relations of the left pulmonary artery:

anterior:	left lung
posterior:	left vagus nerve
	descending aorta
	left main bronchus
superior:	ligamentum arteriosum
	aortic arch
inferior:	left superior pulmonary vein
	left main bronchus

Methods of imaging the pulmonary trunk:

radiographic: plain films and tomography
computed tomography
pulmonary arteriography

radionuclide: ^{99m}Tc-labelled red cell first-pass
studies

THE BRACHIOCEPHALIC ARTERY

The brachiocephalic artery is the first branch of the aortic arch and lies partly in the neck and partly in the superior mediastinum (Fig. 5.27). It ascends behind the manubrium and divides into the right common carotid and subclavian arteries behind the right sternoclavicular joint. It is 5 cm long.

Relations (Figs. 1.7, 1.8):

anterior:	manubrium
	left brachiocephalic vein
	thymus
posterior:	trachea
right:	right brachiocephalic vein
	superior vena cava
	right lung
left:	left common carotid artery
	left brachiocephalic vein

Methods of imaging the brachiocephalic artery:

radiographic: plain films and tomography
computed tomography
arch aortography

THE BRACHIOCEPHALIC VEINS

Each brachiocephalic vein is formed from the union of the subclavian vein and the internal jugular vein (Figs. 1.7, 5.28). It lies partly in the neck and partly in the superior mediastinum. The right brachiocephalic vein descends in front of the brachiocephalic artery, separated from the right lung by pleura. The left brachiocephalic vein is more horizontal, descending in front of the left subclavian and common carotid arteries and behind the manubrium. It is in contact with the parietal pleurae of both lungs. The right vein is 3 cm long; the left is 5 cm long.

THE SUPERIOR VENA CAVA

The superior vena cava drains venous blood from the head, neck and upper limbs to the heart. It is formed in the superior mediastinum from the union of the two brachiocephalic veins behind the manubrium, and the azygos vein drains into it from behind. It enters the right atrium at approximately the level of T7 with its distal part enveloped in pericardium. The superior vena cava has no valves. It is 7 cm long.

Relations (Figs. 1.8–1.10, 1.17):

anterior:	manubrium
	right lung
posterior:	trachea
	azygos vein
	right pulmonary artery
	right superior pulmonary vein
right:	right phrenic nerve
	right lung
left:	brachiocephalic artery
	ascending aorta

Methods of imaging the superior vena cava:

radiographic:	plain films and tomography
	computed tomography
	superior vena cavography

ultrasonographic:	real-time B-mode
	Doppler

THE AZYGOS VENOUS SYSTEM

The azygos and hemiazygos system of veins drains blood from both sides of the diaphragm to the heart. It commences in front of and slightly to the right of L2, from the union of the right subcostal, ascending lumbar and lumbar azygos veins (Fig. 1.21). It ascends, piercing the right crus of the diaphragm, to enter the posterior mediastinum. It continues to ascend to the right of the vertebral column, thoracic duct and aorta, covered by parietal pleura. At the

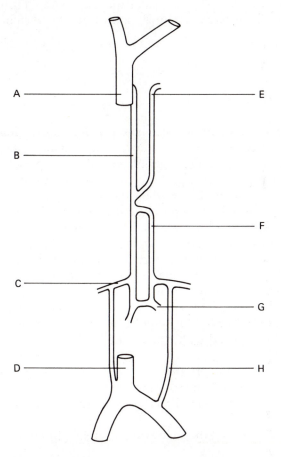

Fig. 1.21 *The azygos venous system*

A: superior vena cava
B: azygos vein
C: subcostal vein
D: inferior vena cava

E: accessory hemiazygos vein
F: hemiazygos vein
G: lumbar azygos vein
H: ascending lumbar vein

level of T5 it arches forward over the right main bronchus and pulmonary artery and enters the superior vena cava (Figs. 1.9, 5.28).

On the left there are two corresponding vessels: the hemiazygos vein inferiorly, which crosses in front of T8 to join the azygos vein and the accessory hemiazygos vein superiorly, which descends to the left of the vertebral column and crosses in front of T7 to join the azygos vein.

Below the diaphragm the azygos venous system forms an alternative drainage to the inferior vena cava. Above, it drains the bronchial veins, posterior intercostal veins (except the uppermost, which drain into the subclavian veins) and mediastinal structures. Throughout its length it has numerous communications with the vertebral venous plexus.

THE DIAPHRAGM

The diaphragm is a dome-shaped sheet which forms the inferior limit of the thoracic cavity. It consists of a central tendon, continuous with the fibrous pericardium, and a peripheral muscular part, contraction of which flattens the dome and increases the intrathoracic volume. The right half is usually higher than the left.

It is attached to the sternum anteriorly and to the costal margin anterolaterally. Posteriorly it is attached to vertebral bodies by crura, muscular slips on either side of the aorta: the right crus attaches to L1–3; the left to L1 and L2. Lateral to the crura the diaphragm is attached to the arcuate ligaments, thickenings of fascia covering psoas and quadratus lumborum muscles.

The diaphragm is pierced by the inferior vena cava at approximately the level of T8, by the oesophagus at the level of T10 and by the aorta and thoracic duct at the level of T12.

Vascular anatomy:

arterial: phrenic arteries   ⎫ arising from the
           posterior intercostal arteries ⎭ thoracic aorta
           inferior phrenic arteries, arising from the abdominal
               aorta
           internal thoracic arteries, arising from the subclavian
               arteries

venous: posterior intercostal veins, draining into the azygos
               venous system
          phrenic veins, draining into the inferior vena cava/
               left renal vein
          internal thoracic veins, draining into the subclavian
               veins

lymph: parasternal nodes
              posterior mediastinal nodes
              para-aortic nodes
              preaortic nodes

Methods of imaging the diaphragm:

radiographic: plain films
                  fluoroscopy
                  computed tomography

ultrasonographic: real-time B-mode

THE BREASTS

The breasts are exocrine organs of lactation. They lie on the deep fascia of the anterior chest wall between the second and sixth ribs. Each is hemispherical in shape with a superolateral prolongation, the axillary tail. The nipple is at its apex.

The breast consists of cells which secrete into lactiferous ducts, each of which opens on to the nipple. Secretory tissue is divided into lobules by connective tissue septa which are continuous with the superficial fascia over the breast. There is no capsule.

The structure of the breast changes with age. It consists largely of duct tissue until the menarche when, under the influence of hormones, secretory tissue develops. This proliferates during pregnancy but atrophies when lactation ceases. With advancing age exocrine tissue is replaced by fat.

Vascular anatomy (Figs. 5.27, 5.28, 7.6, 7.7):
    arterial: internal thoracic artery
                  branches of the axillary artery
                  intercostal arteries

    venous: internal thoracic veins
                  tributaries of the axillary vein
                  intercostal veins

    lymph: axillary nodes
                  parasternal nodes
                  deep cervical nodes

Methods of imaging the breast:

radiographic: mammography
                  double-dye mammography
                  computed tomography

ultrasonographic: real-time B-mode

The abdomen is the part of the body between the thorax and the pelvis. It is a cavity limited by the abdominal wall anteriorly and laterally, by the spinal musculature posteriorly and by the diaphragm superiorly. Inferiorly the abdominal and pelvic cavities are in continuity.

THE STOMACH

The stomach is a hollow, distensible organ which serves as a reservoir for food. It lies in the upper anterior part of the abdominal cavity, mostly to the left of the midline. It has anterior and posterior surfaces which join to form the lesser curve on the right and the greater curve on the left. It consists of the body, capped superiorly by the fundus and continuous inferiorly with the antrum (Fig. 2.1). The body and the antrum are demarcated by the incisura, which is an angulation of the lesser curve. Food enters the stomach from the oesophagus via the cardiac orifice, on the lesser curve at the junction between the fundus and the body. It passes into the duodenum from the antrum via the narrow pyloric canal, a muscular sphincter.

The stomach is enveloped in peritoneum, which supports it. It is suspended from the inferior surface of the liver by the lesser omentum, a double layer of peritoneum which separates at the lesser curve to envelop the stomach and rejoins at the greater curve to form the greater omentum. Superiorly the greater omentum continues as the gastrosplenic ligament.

The stomach wall consists of two muscular layers lined by mucosa which is thrown into folds when the stomach is empty.

Relations (Figs. 2.6–2.9):

    anterior: liver
                     diaphragm
                     anterior abdominal wall

posterior: lesser sac
diaphragm
spleen
splenic vessels
left kidney
left adrenal gland
pancreas
transverse mesocolon
transverse colon

superior: lesser omentum
right and left gastric vessels

inferior: greater omentum
right and left gastroepiploic vessels

Vascular anatomy:
arterial: right and left gastric arteries
right and left gastroepiploic arteries
short gastric arteries, arising from the splenic artery

venous: right and left gastric veins ⎫ draining into
right and left gastroepiploic veins ⎬ the portal vein
short gastric veins ⎭

lymph: hepatic nodes
coeliac nodes

Methods of imaging the stomach:

radiographic: plain films
double-contrast barium meal
computed tomography
coeliac axis arteriography

ultrasonographic: real-time B-mode
endoscopic

radionuclide: gastric emptying studies

THE DUODENUM

The duodenum is a tubular structure forming the proximal part of the small bowel. It is divided into four parts encircling the head of the pancreas (Fig. 2.1). The first part commences at the pyloric canal and is 5 cm long. It is dilated proximally to form the duodenal cap and is directed upward, backward and to the right. The second part descends to the right of the midline and is 8 cm long. The third part crosses the midline horizontally at the level of L3 and is 10 cm long. The fourth part ascends to the left of the midline for 3 cm before curving forward as the duodenojejunal flexure.

The proximal 2 cm of the first part is enveloped in peritoneum which is reflected off the posterior abdominal wall. The duodeno-jejunal flexure is similarly enveloped as it arches forward; superiorly this forms the suspensory ligament of Treitz, a short triangular mesentery. The remainder of the duodenum is retroperitoneal.

The duodenum consists of two muscular layers lined by mucosa which is raised to form valvulae conniventes, circular circumferential folds. The ampulla of Vater, containing the terminations of the common bile duct and the pancreatic duct, is on the medial wall of the second part of the duodenum.

Relations (Figs. 2.8. 2.9):

first part –
    anterolateral: gallbladder
                     liver

    posteromedial: gastroduodenal artery
                     portal vein
                     common bile duct
                     lesser sac
                     head of the pancreas

    superior: hepatic artery ⎫ in the free edge
                portal vein   ⎬ of the
                common bile duct ⎭ lesser omentum
                epiploic foramen
                caudate process of the liver

second part –
>   anterior: liver
>   transverse mesocolon
>   transverse colon
>   small bowel
>
>   posteromedial: common bile duct
>   head of the pancreas
>   inferior vena cava
>   pancreaticoduodenal vessels
>
>   posterolateral: right adrenal gland
>   right kidney

third part –
>   anterior: superior mesenteric vessels
>   root of the small bowel mesentery
>   small bowel
>
>   posterior: right ureter
>   right psoas
>   right gonadal vessels
>   inferior vena cava
>   aorta
>   inferior mesenteric artery

fourth part –
>   anteromedial: root of the small bowel mesentery
>   small bowel
>
>   posterolateral: left renal vessels
>   left gonadal vessels
>   inferior mesenteric vein
>   left kidney
>   left ureter
>   left psoas
>
>   superior: body of the pancreas

Vascular anatomy:

arterial: pancreaticoduodenal arteries

venous: pancreaticoduodenal veins, draining into the portal
vein

lymph: pyloric nodes
pancreaticoduodenal nodes
coeliac nodes

Methods of imaging the duodenum:

radiographic: plain films
double-contrast barium meal
hypotonic duodenography
computed tomography
coeliac axis arteriography
superior mesenteric arteriography

ultrasonographic: real-time B-mode
endoscopic

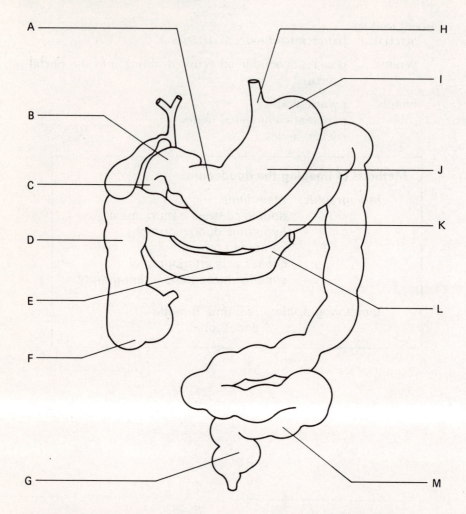

Fig. 2.1 *Arrangement of the stomach, duodenum and colon*

A: antrum of the stomach
B: first part of the
        duodenum
C: second part of the
        duodenum
D: ascending colon
E: third part of the
        duodenum
F: caecum
G: rectum

H: oesophagus
I: fundus of the stomach
J: body of the stomach
K: transverse colon
L: fourth part of the
        duodenum
M: sigmoid colon

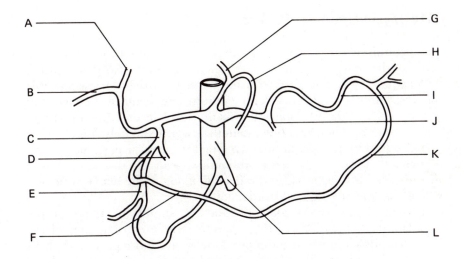

Fig. 2.2 *The coeliac axis*

A: left hepatic artery
B: right hepatic artery
C: gastroduodenal artery
D: right gastric artery
E: superior pancreatico-
    duodenal artery
F: right gastroepiploic artery

G: oesophageal artery
H: left gastric artery
I: splenic artery
J: dorsal pancreatic artery
K: left gastroepiploic artery
L: superior mesenteric
    artery

THE JEJUNUM AND ILEUM

The jejunum is the proximal two fifths, and the ileum the distal three fifths, of the remaining small bowel, there being no clear demarcation between the two. Together with the duodenum they are responsible for absorption of nutrients. The jejunum and ileum are coiled and occupy most of the free space between viscera in the abdominal and pelvic cavities. Their combined length is approximately 5 m.

The jejunum and ileum are enveloped in visceral peritoneum and suspended from the posterior abdominal wall by the small bowel mesentery. This has a parietal reflection along a line between the left side of L2 and the right sacroiliac joint.

The muscular layers and mucosa are similar to those of the duodenum. The calibre of the jejunum is greater than that of the ileum and its circumferential mucosal folds are more pronounced. In 2% of the population a Meckel's diverticulum opens into the distal ileum.

Posterior relations of the small bowel mesentery:

> fourth part of the duodenum
> aorta
> inferior vena cava
> right gonadal vessels
> right ureter
> right psoas

Vascular anatomy:

arterial:	superior mesenteric artery
venous:	superior mesenteric vein, draining into the portal vein
lymph:	mesenteric nodes preaortic nodes

> **Methods of imaging the jejunum and ileum:**
>
> *radiographic:* plain films
> small bowel meal
> small bowel enema
> computed tomography
> superior mesenteric arteriography
>
> *ultrasonographic:* real-time B-mode
>
> *radionuclide:* ^{99m}Tc-pertechnetate Meckel's
> scintigraphy

THE LARGE BOWEL

The large bowel is the distal part of the alimentary canal and conveys the waste products of digestion from the small bowel to the anus. It plays a large part in water resorption. The terminal ileum opens into the posteromedial wall of the caecum via the ileocaecal valve, two crescentic folds of mucosa. The appendix is a diverticulum opening into the caecum below the ileocaecal valve. The caecum continues as the colon, which is divided into three parts (Fig. 2.1): the ascending colon ascends in the right paravertebral gutter as far as its hepatic flexure and is 15 cm long; the descending colon descends in the left paravertebral gutter from its splenic flexure to the sigmoid colon and is 25 cm long; the transverse colon links the two flexures, crossing the midline, and is 50 cm long. (For the sigmoid colon refer to Chapter 3.)

The caecum is enveloped in peritoneum which is reflected off the posterior abdominal wall. The transverse colon is attached to the posterior abdominal wall by the transverse mesocolon, a double layer of peritoneum which separates to envelop it and which has a parietal reflection crossing the posterior abdominal wall between the two flexures. The remaining colon is covered on its front and sides only and peritoneum thus forms medial and lateral paracolic gutters.

Like the proximal alimentary canal, the colon has two muscular coats lined by mucosa. The outer, longitudinal coat is thickened into three teniae coli, muscular bands which run the length of the large bowel. The mucosa is raised into haustra, circular circumferential folds, less numerous than in the small bowel.

Relations:
  caecum –
    anterior: small bowel

    posterior: gonadal vessels
             psoas
             iliacus

  ascending colon –
    anterior: small bowel

    posterior: iliacus
             quadratus lumborum
             right kidney

  transverse colon –
    anterosuperior: liver
                   gallbladder
                   stomach
                   greater omentum
                   spleen

    inferoposterior: small bowel
                   second part of the duodenum
                   head of the pancreas

  descending colon –
    anterior: small bowel

    posterior: diaphragm
             left kidney
             quadratus lumborum
             iliacus
             psoas

Vascular anatomy:
    arterial: superior mesenteric artery – this supplies the
                  proximal large bowel as far as halfway along the
                  transverse colon
              inferior mesenteric artery – this supplies most of the
                  remaining large bowel

    venous: superior mesenteric vein } draining into the
              inferior mesenteric vein } portal vein

    lymph: mesenteric nodes
              preaortic nodes

Methods of imaging the large bowel:

radiographic: plain films
double-contrast barium enema
peroral pneumocolon
computed tomography
superior mesenteric arteriography
inferior mesenteric arteriography

ultrasonographic: endosonic

radionuclide: ^{99m}Tc-labelled red cells, to locate a
point of gastrointestinal
haemorrhage

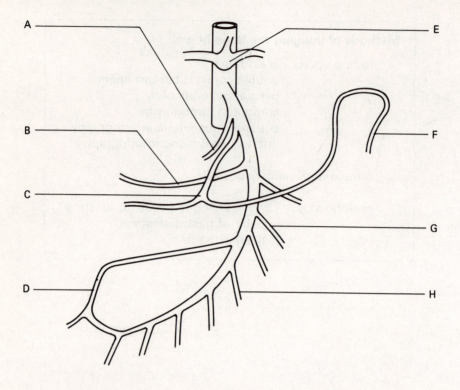

Fig. 2.3   *The superior mesenteric artery*

A: inferior pancreatico-
       duodenal artery
B: right colic artery
C: middle colic artery
D: ileocolic artery

E: coeliac axis
F: anastomosis with inferior
       mesenteric vessels
G: jejunal artery
H: ileal artery

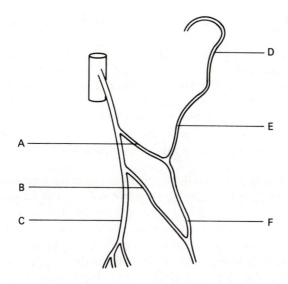

Fig. 2.4   *The inferior mesenteric artery*

A: left colic artery
B: sigmoid artery
C: superior rectal artery

D: anastomosis with
       superior mesenteric
       vessels
E: ascending branch of the
       left colic artery
F: descending branch of the
       left colic artery

THE LIVER

The liver is the largest organ of the body. It has metabolic, endocrine and lymphoid functions and is responsible for the formation of bile. It lies in the right hypochondrium. It has a convex diaphragmatic surface anterosuperiorly and a flat visceral surface facing downward, medially and backward. The interlobar fissure divides the liver into anatomical left and right lobes. It forms a longitudinal groove on the visceral surface which contains the ligamentum teres and the ligamentum venosum, remnants of the umbilical vein and ductus venosus, respectively. The porta hepatis is a transverse groove on the visceral surface of the right lobe, traversed by the portal vein, hepatic artery and common bile duct (Fig. 2.5) and containing lymph nodes.

The liver is covered, on most of its surface, by peritoneum. Reflections of the visceral peritoneum off the diaphragmatic surface form ligaments which suspend the liver from the diaphragm and the abdominal wall. The left and right triangular ligaments are double layers of peritoneum supporting the left and right lobes, respectively; the layers of the right triangular ligament separate medially, becoming the coronary ligament and enclosing a bare area where the liver is directly in contact with the diaphragm. The falciform ligament is a double layer of peritoneum in the midline. Its parietal reflection extends from the diaphragm to the umbilicus and is sickle-shaped. The ligamentum teres runs in its free inferior border. On the visceral surface the peritoneum forms a reflection around the porta hepatis which is continuous with the free edge of the lesser omentum.

The liver consists of hepatocytes and reticuloendothelial cells arranged in lobules, each having a central systemic vein and peripheral portal triads, which consist of branches of the hepatic artery and portal vein and a bile ductule. The central veins unite to form the right, middle and left hepatic veins, which converge on the bare area of the diaphragmatic surface, with the middle hepatic vein running in an avascular plane between the embryological left and right lobes. The portal triads converge on the porta hepatis. The liver has a thin connective tissue capsule.

Relations (Figs. 2.6–2.9):

diaphragmatic:	diaphragm
	right adrenal gland
	inferior vena cava
visceral – left lobe:	aorta
	oesophagus
	stomach
	lesser omentum
	pancreas

visceral – right lobe: duodenum
                                gallbladder
                                right kidney
                                colon

Vascular anatomy:

arterial: hepatic arteries

venous: hepatic veins, draining into the inferior vena cava

portal venous: portal vein, draining the portal system

lymph: portal nodes
               coeliac nodes
               inferior vena caval nodes
               paracardial nodes

Methods of imaging the liver:

radiographic: plain films and tomography
                          computed tomography
                          hepatic arteriography
                          portal venography

ultrasonographic: real-time B-mode (the liver
                                  provides an 'acoustic
                                  window' for imaging other
                                organs)

radionuclide: ^{99m}Tc-labelled colloid scintigraphy
                         ^{67}Ga citrate scintigraphy

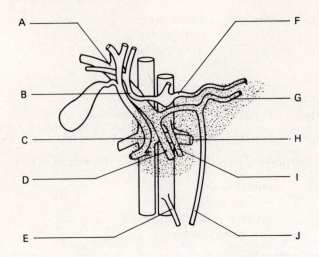

Fig. 2.5   *Arrangement of vessels behind the pancreas*

A: portal vein
B: hepatic artery
C: common bile duct
D: superior mesenteric vein
E: inferior mesenteric artery

F: splenic artery
G: splenic vein
H: renal vein
I: superior mesenteric
        artery
J: inferior mesenteric vein

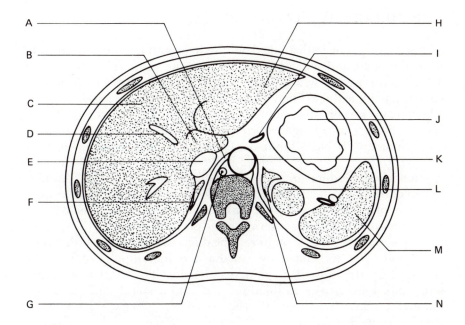

Fig. 2.6 *Cross section through the abdomen at the level of T12*

A: right crus of the
    diaphragm
B: caudate lobe of the liver
C: right lobe of the liver
D: hepatic vein
E: inferior vena cava
F: right adrenal gland
G: cisterna chyli

H: left lobe of the liver
I: left gastric artery
J: stomach
K: aorta
L: left kidney
M: spleen
N: left adrenal gland

THE BILIARY SYSTEM

The biliary system drains bile from the liver into the duodenum. Bile from the right and left lobes drains into the right and left hepatic ducts, respectively, which unite at the porta hepatis to form the common hepatic duct (Fig. 2.5). The gallbladder is a pear-shaped sac which concentrates and stores bile. It is loosely attached to the visceral surface of the right lobe of the liver and is covered elsewhere by peritoneum. It has a fundus, a body and a neck which opens into the cystic duct. The cystic duct is 3 cm long and unites with the common hepatic duct to form the common bile duct. The common bile duct descends in the free edge of the lesser omentum and through the head of the pancreas to the ampulla of Vater. In the free edge of the lesser omentum it lies anterior to the portal vein and to the right of the hepatic artery. It is 8 cm long. The ducts and the gallbladder have a fibromuscular wall lined by mucosa and the ampulla of Vater is encircled by the muscular sphincter of Oddi. The mucosa is raised into small folds in the gallbladder and into a spiral fold along the cystic duct; elsewhere it is smooth.

Relations of the gallbladder (Figs. 2.8, 2.9):

anterior:	abdominal wall
superior:	right lobe of the liver
posteroinferior:	second part of the duodenum transverse colon

Vascular anatomy:

arterial:	hepatic arteries cystic artery, arising from the right hepatic artery
venous:	hepatic veins cystic veins, draining into the portal vein
lymph:	as for the liver, p.55

Methods of imaging the biliary system:

radiographic: plain films and tomography
oral cholecystography
intravenous cholangiography
percutaneous transhepatic
  cholangiography
endoscopic retrograde
  cholangiography
operative cholangiography
postoperative T-tube
  cholangiography
computed tomography

ultrasonographic: real-time B-mode
endoscopic

radionuclide: radioiodine-HIDA scintigraphy

THE SPLEEN

The spleen is a lymphoid and haemopoietic organ. It lies posteriorly in the left hypochondrium overlying the ninth, tenth and eleventh ribs. It has a convex diaphragmatic surface on the left and a visceral surface facing downward, forward and to the right. The diaphragmatic and visceral surfaces meet at the superior border, which has a notch, and the inferior border. The spleen has anterior and posterior extremities and a maximum length of 12 cm. The splenic vessels enter the spleen at the hilum, on its visceral surface.

The spleen is almost entirely covered by peritoneum. On its visceral surface reflections form the gastrosplenic ligament anteriorly and the lienorenal ligament posteriorly. The gastrosplenic ligament is continuous with the greater omentum and the lienorenal ligament contains the tail of the pancreas and the splenic vessels.

The spleen consists of lymphoid cells, lymph vessels and venous sinusoids supported by a network of fibroelastic trabeculae and contained within a fibroelastic capsule.

Visceral relations:

> stomach
> left kidney
> left adrenal gland
> tail of the pancreas
> colon

Vascular anatomy (Figs. 2.2, 2.3):

arterial:	splenic artery
venous:	splenic vein, draining into the portal vein
lymph:	pancreaticosplenic nodes
	coeliac nodes

Methods of imaging the spleen:

radiographic: plain films and tomography
computed tomography
coeliac axis arteriography

ultrasonographic: real-time B-mode

radionuclide: ^{99m}Tc-labelled colloid scintigraphy
^{99m}Tc-labelled damaged red cells

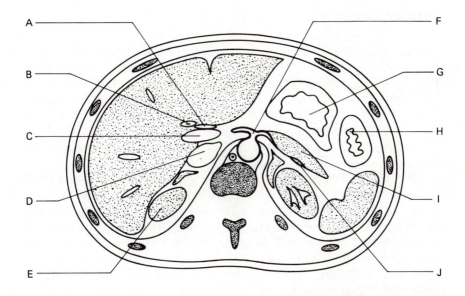

Fig. 2.7 *Cross section through the abdomen at the level of T12/L1*

A: hepatic artery
B: common hepatic duct
C: portal vein
D: inferior vena cava
E: right kidney

F: coeliac axis
G: stomach
H: splenic flexure of the
    colon
I: body of the pancreas
J: splenic artery

THE PANCREAS

The pancreas is a gland with both endocrine and exocrine functions, the latter concerned with digestion. It is a retroperitoneal organ lying on the posterior abdominal wall, on either side of the midline, in the loop formed by the duodenum. It consists of a head, neck, body and tail (Fig. 2.5). The head lies to the right of the midline and its inferior uncinate process projects to the left. The neck, body and tail are directed upward and to the left, with some of the tail lying in the lienorenal ligament. It is 15 cm long.

The exocrine cells of the pancreas are arranged in lobules and drain their products into interlobular ducts which unite to form the main pancreatic duct. This unites with the common bile duct in the ampulla of Vater. The accessory duct drains the uncinate process and dorsal part of the head of the pancreas into the duodenum via an accessory opening 3 cm proximal to the ampulla of Vater. The endocrine cells are arranged in islets dispersed throughout the pancreatic substance.

Relations (Figs. 2.7–2.9):

> head –
>> anterior: first part of the duodenum
>>> lesser sac
>>> transverse colon
>>> small bowel
>>
>> posterior: common bile duct
>>> inferior vena cava
>>> right renal vein
>>
>> right: second part of the duodenum
>>
>> inferior: third part of the duodenum

> uncinate process –
>> anterior: *superior mesenteric vessels
>>
>> posterior: left renal vein
>>
>> inferior: third part of the duodenum

> neck –
>> anterior: gastroduodenal artery
>>> pancreaticoduodenal vessels
>>> lesser sac
>>> stomach

posterior: portal vein
             *superior mesenteric vessels

body –
    anterior: lesser sac
                stomach
                transverse colon
                small bowel

    posterior: aorta
                 splenic vein
                 inferior mesenteric vein
                 diaphragm
                 left adrenal gland
                 left kidney

    superior: coeliac axis
                splenic artery

    inferior: duodenojejunal flexure

tail –
    lateral: hilum of the spleen

Vascular anatomy:
    arterial: pancreaticoduodenal arteries
                splenic artery

    venous: pancreaticoduodenal veins ⎫   draining into the
              splenic vein   ⎬   portal vein
                                        ⎭

    lymph: pancreaticosplenic nodes
             preaortic nodes

Methods of imaging the pancreas:

radiographic: plain films and tomography
                  computed tomography
                  endoscopic retrograde
                      pancreatography

ultrasonographic: real-time B-mode
                      endoscopic

---

* Note that the superior mesenteric vessels are posterior to the head but anterior to the uncinate process.

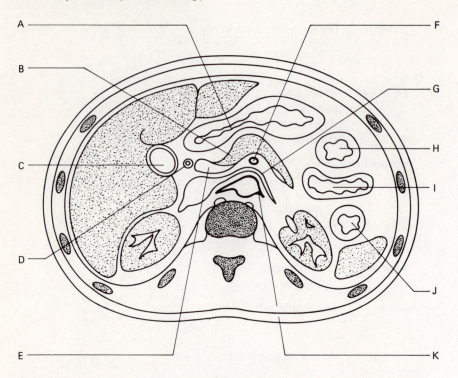

Fig. 2.8 *Cross section through the abdomen at the level of L1/2*

A: pylorus
B: neck of the pancreas
C: gallbladder
D: common bile duct
E: splenic/superior
    mesenteric venous
    confluence

F: superior mesenteric
    artery
G: left renal vein
H: transverse colon
I: jejunum
J: descending colon
K: left renal artery

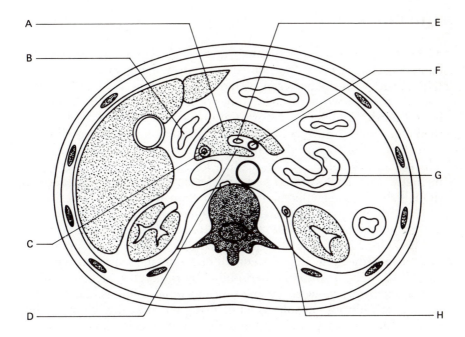

Fig. 2.9 *Cross section through the abdomen at the level of L2*

A: head of the pancreas
B: duodenum
C: common bile duct
D: uncinate process of the pancreas

E: superior mesenteric vein
F: superior mesenteric artery
G: duodenojejunal flexure
H: left ureter

THE KIDNEYS

The kidneys are excretory organs which regulate fluid and electrolyte balance. They are retroperitoneal structures, lying in the paravertebral gutters on the posterior wall of the abdomen. Each kidney has anterior and posterior surfaces, superior and inferior poles, a convex lateral border and a concave medial border. The renal vessels enter the kidney, and the ureter arises from it, at the hilum. The right hilum is at the level of L2 and the left hilum is at the level of the L1/2 disc. The kidneys lie obliquely so that their long axes are directed upward, medially and backward. They are 12 cm long and 6 cm across, though the left is usually slightly larger than the right.

The kidneys, their vessels and the upper ureters, together with the adrenal glands and perirenal fat-pads, are enclosed in renal fascia.

The kidney consists of a central medulla whose conical pyramids project into the collecting system to form cup-shaped minor calyces (Fig. 2.10). The medulla is surrounded by the cortex, some of which extends centrally between the pyramids as renal columns. The kidney has a tough fibrous capsule which is invaginated at the hilum by the pelvis of the ureter posteriorly and the renal vessels anteriorly. The three or four major tributaries of the pelvis are known as major calyces. The renal sinus is the space between the renal substance and the collecting system, and contains fat.

The functional unit of the kidney is the uriniferous tubule, which consists of a renal corpuscle in the cortex, where filtration occurs, and a renal tubule in the medulla, where secretion and resorption occur. The uriniferous tubules unite to form collecting tubules which open on to the apex of a pyramid.

Relations of the right kidney (Figs. 2.6–2.9):

anterior:	liver
	duodenum
	colon
	small bowel
posterior:	diaphragm
	psoas
	quadratus lumborum
	transversus abdominis
	subcostal vessels
superior:	adrenal gland
medial:	renal vessels
	ureter
	inferior vena cava

Relations of the left kidney (Figs. 2.7–2.9):

    anterior: spleen
                    stomach
                    body of the pancreas
                    small bowel
                    colon

    posterior: as for right kidney, opposite

    medial: adrenal gland
                    renal vessels
                    aorta
                    ureter

Vascular anatomy:

    arterial: renal artery

    venous: renal vein

    lymph: para-aortic nodes

Methods of imaging the kidneys:

    radiographic: plain films and tomography
                           intravenous urography
                           antegrade pyelography
                           retrograde pyelography
                           computed tomography
                           arteriography

    ultrasonographic: real-time B-mode

    radionuclide: ^{99m}Tc-DMSA static scintigraphy
                      ^{99m}Tc-DTPA dynamic scintigraphy
                      radioiodine-hippuran dynamic
                           scintigraphy

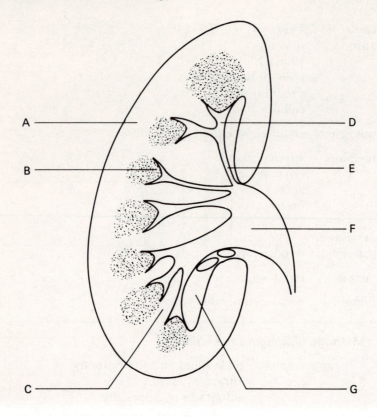

Fig. 2.10 *The structure of the kidney*

A: cortex
B: medullary pyramid
C: column

D: minor calyx
E: major calyx
F: pelvis of the ureter
G: sinus

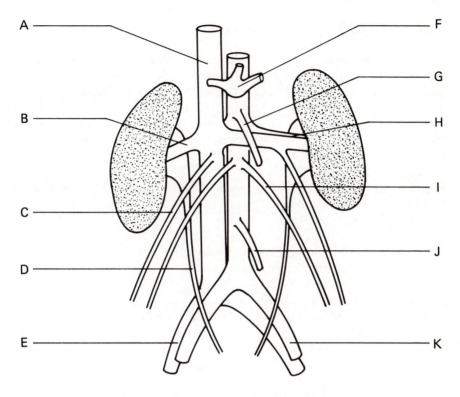

Fig. 2.11 *Structures on the posterior abdominal wall*

A: inferior vena cava
B: renal vein
C: gonadal vein
D: ureter
E: common iliac vein

F: coeliac axis
G: superior mesenteric artery
H: renal artery
I: gonadal artery
J: inferior mesenteric artery
K: common iliac artery

THE URETERS

The ureters are muscular tubes which drain urine from the kidneys to the bladder. They are retroperitoneal structures, half in the abdomen and half in the pelvis. Each ureter commences as the renal pelvis and descends, initially enclosed in renal fascia, to the pelvis, in front of the sacroiliac joint. In the pelvis the ureter lies in the pelvic fascia, curving forward and medially on levator ani to enter the bladder at its lateral angle. Each ureter is 25 cm long.

The ureter consists of muscular layers within a fibrous coat. It is lined by mucosa which is continuous with that of the bladder and that covering the renal papillae.

Relations of the right ureter:
abdominal –
anterior: second part of the duodenum
right colic vessels
ileocolic vessels
gonadal vessels (Fig. 2.11)
root of the small bowel mesentery

pelvic (Figs. 3.2, 4.1, 4.2) –
anterosuperior: vas deferens (male)
broad ligament ⎫
uterine artery   ⎬ (female)
ovary   ⎭

posterior: psoas
common iliac vessels (Fig. 2.11)
sacroiliac joint
levator ani

medial: seminal vesicle (male)
lateral fornix (female)

Relations of the left ureter:
abdominal –
anterior: left colic vessels
gonadal vessels (Fig. 2.11)
sigmoid mesocolon

pelvic (Figs. 3.2, 4.1, 4.2) –

  anterosuperior: as for the right ureter, opposite

  posterior: as for the right ureter, opposite

  medial: ~~abdominal aorta~~
        seminal vesicle (male)
        lateral fornix (female)

Vascular anatomy:

  arterial: renal artery
        gonadal artery
        branches from the aorta
        internal iliac artery
        vesical arteries
        uterine artery

  venous: renal vein
        gonadal vein
        internal iliac vein
        vesical veins
        uterine vein

  lymph: para-aortic nodes
        common iliac nodes
        internal iliac nodes
        external iliac nodes

Methods of imaging the ureter:

  radiographic: plain films and tomography
            intravenous urography
            antegrade pyelography
            retrograde pyelography
            micturating cystography
            computed tomography

  ultrasonographic: real-time B-mode

  radionuclide: ^{99m}Tc-DTPA dynamic scintigraphy
            radioiodine-hippuran dynamic
              scintigraphy

THE ADRENAL GLANDS

The adrenal glands are endrocrine organs on the posterior abdominal wall, in close relation to the superior poles of the kidneys. Seen from the front, the right gland is triangular, with its base on the antero-superior surface of the kidney, and the left gland is crescentic, with its concave surface extending down the superomedial border of the kidney as far as the hilum. In transverse section the glands are 'Y-shaped', each having an anterior limb, a posteromedial limb and a posterolateral limb.

The adrenal glands are enclosed in renal fascia and the left gland is retroperitoneal.

The gland consists of a central medulla concerned with secretion of adrenergic hormones and a peripheral cortex concerned with secretion of steroid hormones. It has a fibrous capsule.

Relations of the right adrenal gland (Figs. 2.6, 2.7):

    anterior: inferior vena cava
                liver

    posteroinferior: kidney

    medial: crus of the diaphragm
                psoas

Relations of the left adrenal gland (Figs. 2.6, 2.7):

    anterior: lesser sac
                stomach
                pancreas

    posterolateral: kidney

    medial: aorta
                crus of the diaphragm
                psoas

Vascular anatomy:

    arterial: inferior phrenic artery
                branches from the aorta
                renal artery

    venous: adrenal vein, draining into the inferior vena cava/left renal vein

    lymph: para-aortic nodes

Methods of imaging the adrenal gland:

radiographic: plain films and tomography
computed tomography
arteriography
venography

ultrasonographic: real-time B-mode

radionuclide: ^{75}Se-cholesterol scintigraphy
radioiodine-MIBG scintigraphy

THE PERITONEUM

The peritoneum is a serous membrane which lines the abdominal and pelvic cavities and forms a covering and a support for the viscera. It contains a potential space, the peritoneal cavity, which usually encloses a small amount of fluid.

The complex folding of the visceral peritoneum divides the peritoneal cavity into the greater and lesser sacs and results in the formation of spaces (Fig. 2.12) where, in disease, fluid or gas may become localized. The lesser sac is a pocket-shaped diverticulum which communicates with the greater sac via the epiploic foramen, at its right extremity. Its posterior wall is formed by parietal peritoneum covering the diaphragm, the body of the pancreas, the left kidney and the left adrenal gland. Its anterior wall is formed by the visceral peritoneum of the lesser omentum, stomach and greater omentum. It is limited by the lesser omentum superiorly and on the right, by the gastrosplenic and lienorenal ligaments on the left and by the greater omentum inferiorly.

The greater sac comprises the remainder of the abdominal and pelvic cavities. Further subdivisions are formed by peritoneal reflections: the left and right subphrenic spaces are between the diaphragm and the respective lobes of the liver; the subhepatic space is between the right lobe of the liver and the right kidney; the right infracolic space is between the transverse mesocolon and the small bowel mesentery; the left infracolic space is between the small bowel mesentery and the sigmoid mesocolon.

The rectovesical pouch is in the male pelvis and the rectouterine pouch is the equivalent space in the female pelvis.

Methods of imaging the peritoneum and peritoneal cavity:

radiographic: plain films
computed tomography

ultrasonographic: real-time B-mode

radionuclide: ^{67}Ga citrate scintigraphy
^{111}In-labelled leucocyte
scintigraphy

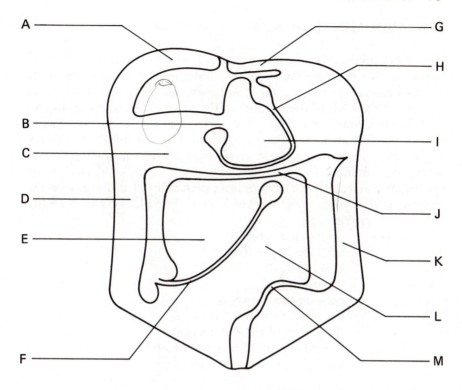

Fig. 2.12 *Peritoneal reflections and spaces*

A: right subphrenic space
B: epiploic foramen
C: subhepatic space
D: right paracolic gutter
E: right infracolic space
F: small bowel mesentery

G: left subphrenic space
H: greater omentum
I: lesser sac
J: transverse mesocolon
K: left paracolic gutter
L: left infracolic space
M: sigmoid mesocolon

THE ABDOMINAL AORTA

The abdominal aorta is the continuation of the descending thoracic aorta on the posterior wall of the abdominal cavity, where it is retroperitoneal. It pierces the diaphragm at the level of T12 and descends to the left of the midline to the level of L4, where it divides into the common iliac arteries. The aorta gives rise, in the midline, to the coeliac axis at the level of T12/L1, the superior mesenteric artery at L1, the inferior mesenteric artery at L3 and the median sacral artery at its bifurcation. The inferior phrenic, middle adrenal, renal and lumbar arteries are branches from each side of the aorta, with the renal arteries arising at the level of L1/2 (Fig. 2.11). It is 12 cm long.
Relations (Figs. 2.6–2.9):

anterior: coeliac axis and branches
            left lobe of the liver
            lesser sac
            splenic vein
            body of the pancreas
            left renal vein
            third part of the duodenum
            root of the small bowel mesentery
            small bowel

posterior: left lumbar veins
            vertebral column
            left psoas

left: left sympathetic trunk
            left crus of the diaphragm
            left adrenal gland
            left ureter
            fourth part of the duodenum

right: cisterna chyli
            azygos vein
            right crus of the diaphragm
            inferior vena cava

Methods of imaging the abdominal aorta:

radiographic: plain films and tomography
                  computed tomography
                  aortography

ultrasonographic: real-time B-mode
                      Doppler

THE INFERIOR VENA CAVA

The inferior vena cava drains venous blood from the lower limbs, pelvis and abdomen to the heart. It is formed from the union of the common iliac veins in front of the body of L5 and ascends on the posterior abdominal wall, to the right of the midline (Fig. 2.11). Its greater part is retroperitoneal but its upper abdominal part is embedded in the posterior surface of the right lobe of the liver and its terminal part lies in the middle mediastinum of the thorax. It drains the lumbar, renal and hepatic veins and the right gonadal, adrenal and phrenic veins. It is connected, via the lumbar azygos or ascending lumbar vein, to the azygos venous system. The inferior vena cava pierces the diaphragm at approximately the level of T8 and its terminal part is enveloped in pericardium. There are no valves in the inferior vena cava except for a semilunar valve where it enters the right atrium. It is 20 cm long.

Relations (Figs. 2.6–2.9, 2.11):

anterior:	right lobe of the liver
	epiploic foramen
	portal vein
	hepatic artery
	common bile duct
	second part of the duodenum
	head of the pancreas
	third part of the duodenum
	right gonadal artery
	root of the small bowel mesentery
	right common iliac artery
posterior:	right adrenal gland
	right inferior phrenic artery
	right adrenal artery
	right renal artery
	right crus of the diaphragm
	vertebral column
	right psoas
right:	right ureter
left:	aorta

Methods of imaging the inferior vena cava: as for the abdominal aorta, opposite

THE PORTAL VEIN

The portal vein drains venous blood from the intestine, biliary system, pancreas and spleen into the liver. It is formed from the union of the superior mesenteric vein and the splenic vein (Fig. 2.13) behind the neck of the pancreas, at the level of the L1/2 disc. It runs upward and to the right in the free edge of the lesser omentum to enter the liver at the porta hepatis, where it divides into right and left branches. It is 8 cm long.

Relations of the portal vein (Figs. 2.5, 2.7, 2.8):

    anterior: hepatic artery

                common bile duct

                neck of the pancreas

    posterior: epiploic foramen

                inferior vena cava

Methods of imaging the portal vein:

    radiographic: computed tomography

                       late-phase superior mesenteric

                           arteriography

                       transhepatic portal venography

                       splenoportography

                       umbilical venography

    ultrasonographic: real-time B-mode

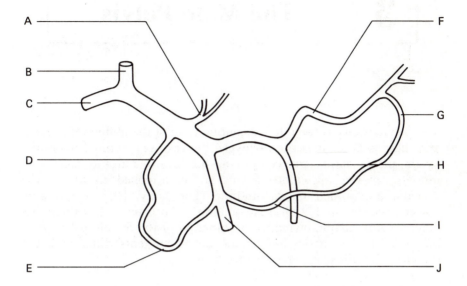

Fig. 2.13 *The portal venous system*

A: gastric veins
B: left branch of the portal vein
C: right branch of the portal vein
D: superior pancreatico-duodenal vein
E: inferior pancreatico-duodenal vein

F: splenic vein
G: left gastroepiploic vein
H: inferior mesenteric vein
I: right gastroepiploic vein
J: superior mesenteric vein

3 | The Male Pelvis

The pelvic cavity is the inferior continuation of the abdominal cavity and there is no demarcation between the two. It is limited inferiorly by the pelvic diaphragm comprising the levator ani and coccygeus muscles, paired musculotendinous sheets attached to the pelvic skeleton and joined in the midline. The bony, ligamentous and muscular skeleton (Fig. 3.1) is common to both sexes, but there are differences in shape, owing to the function of the female pelvis as a birth canal. The male and female pelvic contents differ and are therefore described in separate chapters.

THE SIGMOID COLON

The sigmoid colon is the part of the large bowel between the descending colon and the rectum. It lies in a variable position in contact with the bladder and loops of small bowel, and is approximately 40 cm long.

It is attached to the posterior and left lateral wall of the pelvic cavity by the sigmoid mesocolon, a double layer of peritoneum which separates to envelop it. The sigmoid mesocolon has a parietal reflection in the shape of an inverted 'V', with the apex overlying the left sacroiliac joint.

Posterior relations of the root of the sigmoid mesocolon:
>bifurcation of the left common iliac artery
>left ureter
>superior rectal vessels
>left psoas

Vascular anatomy (Fig. 2.4):

arterial:	sigmoid arteries, arising from the inferior mesenteric artery
venous:	sigmoid veins, draining into the inferior mesenteric vein
lymph:	preaortic nodes

Methods of imaging the sigmoid colon:

radiographic: plain films and tomography
double-contrast barium enema
computed tomography
inferior mesenteric arteriography

radionuclide: ^{99m}Tc-labelled red cells may be used
to locate a point of
gastrointestinal haemorrhage

THE RECTUM

The rectum is the part of the large bowel beyond the sigmoid mesocolon. It commences in front of the body of S3 and terminates 3 cm in front of the coccyx, as the rectal ampulla. It follows the anteroposterior curve of the sacrum as far as the perineal flexure, a sharp backward curve which marks the anorectal junction. Seen from the front, the rectum has a variable 'S' shape. It is 12 cm long.

The lowest third of the rectum is entirely embedded in the pelvic fascia. The middle third is covered by peritoneum on its front only and the uppermost third is enveloped by peritoneum on its front and sides. Peritoneum thus forms paired pararectal fossae lateral to the uppermost third and a single rectovesical pouch anterior to the upper two thirds of the male rectum. The pararectal fossae contain loops of small bowel and sigmoid colon.

The mucosa lining the rectum is raised into circumferential folds similar to those in the colon but incomplete, having a crescentic rather than a circular shape.

Relations (Figs. 3.3, 3.5):

anterior: rectovesical pouch
bladder
ampullae of the vasa deferentia
seminal vesicles
ejaculatory ducts
prostate gland

posterior: superior rectal vessels
sacral vessels
sympathetic chain + lumbosacral
sacrum and coccyx

lateral: piriformis
             coccygeus
             levator ani

Vascular anatomy (Figs. 2.4, 3.6):
    arterial: superior rectal artery, arising from the inferior
                  mesenteric artery
                  middle rectal arteries
                  inferior rectal arteries

    venous: rectal plexus, draining into the inferior mesenteric
                  and internal iliac veins

    lymph: pararectal nodes
                 preaortic nodes
                 internal iliac nodes

Methods of imaging the rectum: as for the sigmoid colon, p.81

THE BLADDER

The bladder is a hollow, distensible, muscular organ which serves as a reservoir for urine. It lies in the anterior pelvis, mostly in the pelvic fascia. When empty it has a pyramidal shape, with a base posteriorly, a neck inferiorly, two inferolateral surfaces and a superior surface. There are two inferolateral surfaces and a superior surface. When full it has a capacity of 300 ml and distends upward into the abdominal cavity, acquiring an ovoid shape. On transverse section, however, it is rectangular.

The male bladder is suspended from the anterior wall of the abdomen by the median umbilical ligament, which is attached to the apex. It is supported on levator ani by the prostate gland and several condensations of the pelvic fascia: paired puboprostatic ligaments anteriorly, paired lateral ligaments between the bladder and the lateral pelvic walls, and a single posterior ligament between the bladder and the rectum.

The bladder is covered superiorly by peritoneum, the anterior reflection of which lies at the level of the pubic symphysis when the bladder is empty but as high as the umbilicus when it is full. The posterior reflection forms the lower limit of the rectovesical pouch in the male.

The bladder is lined by mucosa, most of which is raised into folds by the contracted muscularis. The mucosa of the bladder base, however, is smooth and forms the trigone. This has a ureteric orifice at each lateral angle and the internal urethral orifice at the inferior angle, which corresponds to the bladder neck.

Relations (Figs. 3.2, 3.3, 3.5):

superior: small bowel
            sigmoid colon

inferolateral: pubic bones
                 levator ani
                 obturator internus

inferior: prostate gland

posterior: ampullae of the vasa deferentia
             seminal vesicles
             rectovesical pouch
             rectum

Vascular anatomy:

arterial: superior vesical arteries
            inferior vesical arteries

venous: vesical plexus, draining into the internal iliac veins

lymph: internal iliac nodes
         external iliac nodes

Methods of imaging the bladder:

radiographic: plain films and tomography
                  intravenous urography
                  micturating cystourethrography
                  retrograde urethrography
                  computed tomography

ultrasonographic: real-time B-mode (the bladder
                      provides an 'acoustic
                      window' for imaging other
                      organs)

radionuclide: ^{99m}Tc-DTPA dynamic renal
                  scintigraphy
                  radioiodine-hippuran dynamic
                  renal scintigraphy

THE PROSTATE GLAND

The prostate gland is an exocrine organ which lies between the neck of the bladder and levator ani, embedded in pelvic fascia. It has the shape of a truncated cone, with the base uppermost. It is 3 cm high and 4 cm in diameter. The gland is traversed vertically by the urethra and, in its upper half, by paired ejaculatory ducts. These open into the posterior wall of the urethra together with 20–30 prostatic ducts and the single orifice of the prostatic utricle, a blind-ended sac.

The prostate gland consists of muscular and secretory cells and has a fibromuscular capsule.

Relations (Figs. 3.4, 3.5):

    superior: bladder

    inferolateral: pubic bones
                    levator ani

    posterior: rectum

Vascular anatomy:

    arterial: inferior vesical arteries
               middle rectal arteries

    venous: prostatic plexus, draining into the internal vertebral plexus
               vesical plexus, draining into the internal iliac veins

    lymph: internal iliac nodes

Methods of imaging the prostate gland:

    radiographic: intravenous urography
                    ascending urethrography
                    computed tomography

    ultrasonographic: real-time B-mode
                       endosonic, via the urethra or rectum

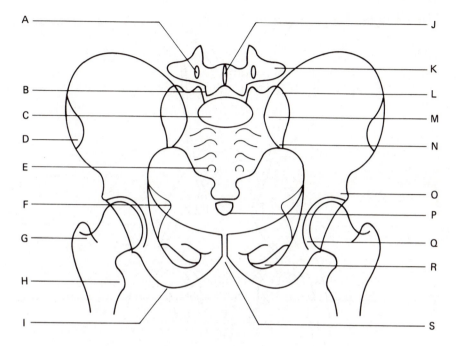

Fig. 3.1 *The pelvic skeleton*

A:	lumbar pedicle	J:	spinous process
B:	facet joint	K:	transverse process
C:	vertebral body	L:	sacroiliac joint
D:	anterior superior iliac spine	M:	posterior superior iliac spine
E:	sacral foramen	N:	posterior inferior iliac spine
F:	ischial spine	O:	anterior inferior iliac spine
G:	greater trochanter	P:	coccyx
H:	lesser trochanter	Q:	acetabular fossa
I:	ischial tuberosity	R:	obturator foramen
		S:	pubic symphysis

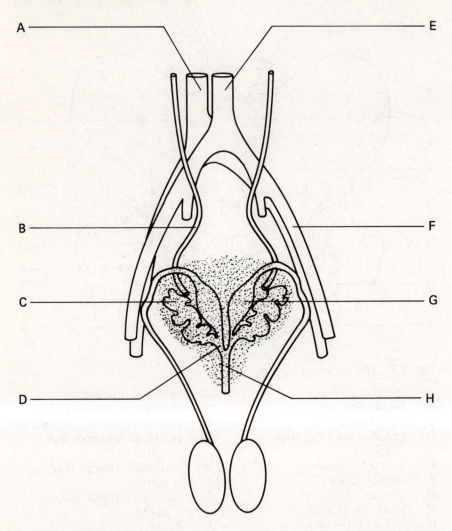

Fig. 3.2 *Structures behind the male bladder*

A: inferior vena cava
B: ureter
C: seminal vesicle
D: ejaculatory duct

E: aorta
F: external iliac artery
G: ampulla of the vas
       deferens
H: urethra

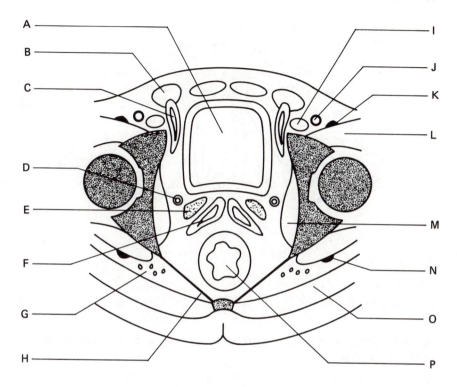

Fig. 3.3 *Cross section through the male pelvis at the level of the ischial spines*

A: bladder
B: spermatic cord
C: vas deferens
D: ureter
E: seminal vesicle
F: ampulla of the vas
    deferens
G: superior and inferior
    gluteal vessels
H: sacrospinous ligament

I: femoral vein
J: femoral artery
K: femoral nerve
L: iliopsoas
M: obturator internus
N: sciatic nerve
O: gluteus maximus
P: rectum

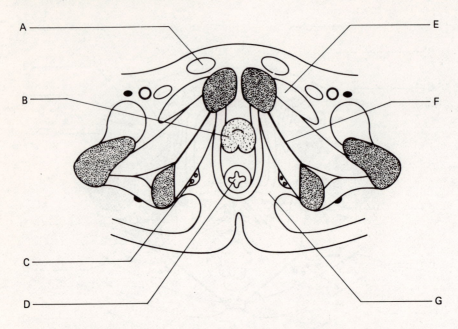

Fig. 3.4 *Cross section through the male pelvis at the level of the pubic symphysis*

A: spermatic cord
B: prostate gland
C: pudendal canal
D: anal canal

E: pectineus
F: obturator membrane
G: ischiorectal fossa

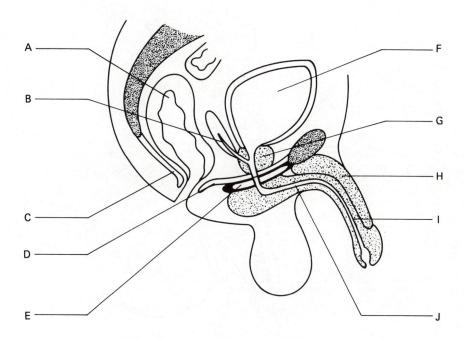

Fig. 3.5 *Sagittal section through the male pelvis*

A: rectum
B: ampulla of the vas
     deferens
C: levator ani
D: levator ani
E: urogenital diaphragm

F: bladder
G: prostate gland
H: corpora cavernosa
I: corpus spongiosum
J: urethra

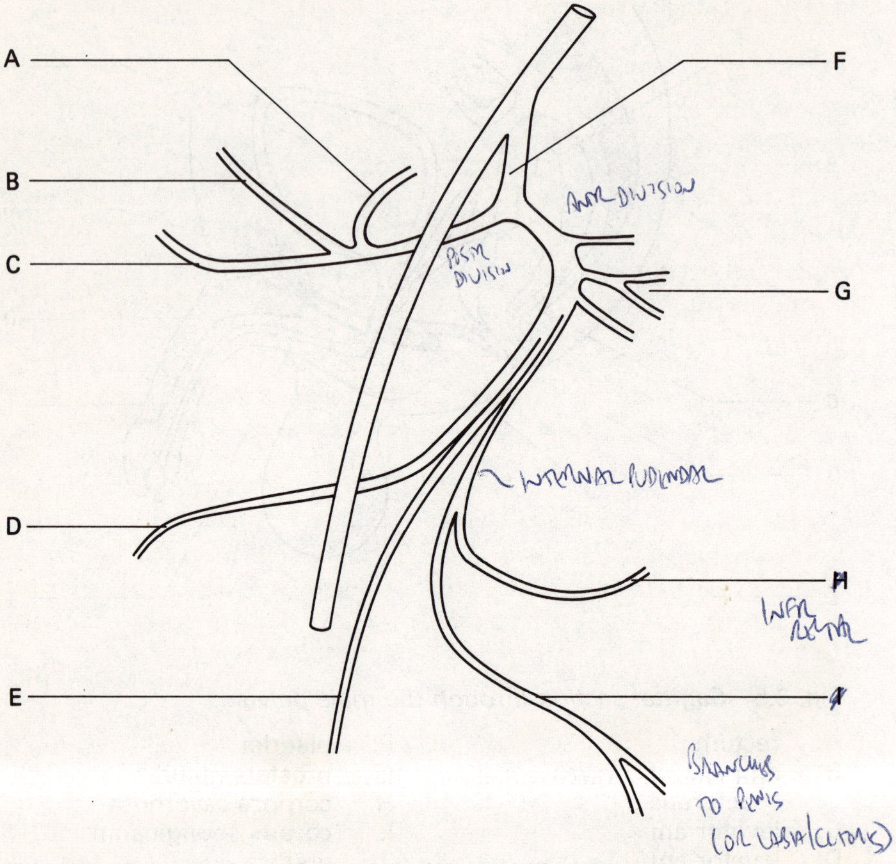
A
B
C
D
E
F
G
H
I
ANTR DIVISION
POSTR DIVISION
INTERNAL PUDENDAL
INFR RECTAL
BRANCHES TO PENIS (OR LABIA/CLITORIS)

Fig. 3.6 *Frontal view of the right internal iliac artery*

A: lateral sacral artery
B: iliolumbar artery
C: superior gluteal artery
D: inferior gluteal artery
E: obturator artery
F: internal iliac artery
G: vesical, uterine and middle rectal arteries
H: inferior rectal artery
I: internal pudendal artery

Middle rectal = ♀ uterine

THE TESTES, EPIDIDYMES AND SPERMATIC CORDS

The testes are reproductive and endocrine organs responsible for the production of sperm. They lie in the scrotum, suspended by the spermatic cord. Each is oval in shape, having medial and lateral surfaces, anterior and posterior borders and superior and inferior poles (Fig. 3.7). Each is 4 cm high and 2.5 cm across.

The testis consists of spermatogenic cells arranged in lobules, supported by fibrous septa which arise from the tunica albuginea, a fibrous capsule. Semen drains in seminiferous tubules to the rete testis, a plexus of vessels in the testis near its posterior border. Efferent ductules pierce the fibrous capsule near the superior pole to convey sperm from the rete testis to the head of the epididymis.

The tunica vaginalis is a serous sac, continuous with the peritoneum in early life and connected to it by the processus vaginalis. It has a parietal layer lining the scrotum and a visceral layer surrounding the anterior part of the testis.

The epididymis is a coiled tube attached to the posterior border of the testis, with its head at the superior pole and its tail at the inferior pole. Sperm pass from the head to the tail and then into the vas deferens, which ascends medial to the epididymis.

The spermatic cord extends from the posterior border of the testis to the deep inguinal ring. It consists of three fascial layers, which are continuous with the oblique and transverse muscles of the abdominal wall, and contains the vas deferens, blood and lymph vessels, nerves and the processus vaginalis.

Vascular anatomy (Fig. 2.11):

    arterial: testicular artery
                  cremasteric artery
                  artery of the vas deferens

    venous: pampiniform plexus, draining via the testicular vein
                  into the inferior vena cava/left renal vein

    lymph: para-aortic nodes

Methods of imaging the testis:

   radiographic: computed tomography

   ultrasonographic: real-time B-mode

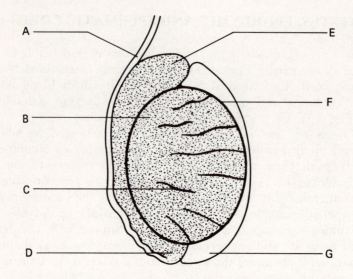

Fig. 3.7   *Oblique parasagittal section through the testis*

A: vas deferens   E: head of the epididymis
B: rete testis   F: tunica albuginea
C: septum   G: tunica vaginalis
D: tail of the epididymis

THE VASA DEFERENTIA

The vasa deferentia are muscular tubes which convey sperm from the epididymis to the ejaculatory ducts. Each vas deferens commences at the tail of the epididymis, in the scrotum. It passes upward in the spermatic cord to the deep inguinal ring, where it separates from other structures of the spermatic cord to pass backward, as an extraperitoneal structure, around the wall of the pelvic cavity to the ischial spine. Here it loops over the ureter and runs forward to the ampulla, its terminal dilatation. This joins the seminal vesicle to form the ejaculatory duct behind the bladder neck. The vas deferens is 45 cm long.

Relations (Figs. 3.2, 3.3):
    scrotum –
        anterior: testis

        lateral: epididymis

spermatic cord –
    anterior: vessels, nerves and the remains of the processus
                vaginalis

pelvic wall –
    medial: inferior epigastric vessels
              pelvic contents

    lateral: external iliac vessels
              branches of the internal iliac vessels
              ureter
              ischial spine

ampulla –
    anterior: bladder

    posterior: rectovesical pouch
              rectum

    lateral: seminal vesicle

Vascular anatomy:
    arterial: testicular artery
              inferior vesical artery
              middle rectal artery

    venous: testicular vein
              vesical plexus, draining into the internal iliac veins

    lymph: para-aortic nodes
              internal iliac nodes

Methods of imaging the vas deferens:

    radiographic: computed tomography
                     vasography

    ultrasonographic: real-time B-mode
                           endosonic

THE EJACULATORY DUCTS AND SEMINAL VESICLES

Each ejaculatory duct is formed by the union of a vas deferens and a seminal vesicle and conducts seminal fluid from these into the prostatic urethra. The ejaculatory duct lies behind the bladder neck, partly in the pelvic fascia and partly in the substance of the prostate gland (Figs. 3.4, 3.5). The seminal vesicle lies behind the posterior wall of the bladder (Figs. 3.2, 3.3), mostly in pelvic fascia but with its tip covered by the peritoneum of the rectovesical pouch. Each ejaculatory duct is 2 cm long and each seminal vesicle is 5 cm long.
Vascular anatomy: as for the bladder, p.83.
Methods of imaging the ejaculatory duct and seminal vesicle: as for the vas deferens, p.93.

THE MALE PERINEUM AND PENIS

The male perineum is a compartment in the lower pelvis lying beneath the pelvic cavity and separated from it by the pelvic diaphragm (Fig.3.5). In transverse section the perineum is diamond-shaped, having the pubic symphysis, coccyx and both ischial tuberosities as vertices. The perineum is divided by a line between the ischial tuberosities into an anterior, urogenital triangle and a posterior, anal triangle.

The urogenital triangle is further divided into superficial and deep pouches by the urogenital diaphragm. This is attached to the pubic bodies anteriorly and to the ischiopubic rami as far back as the ischial tuberosities, having a free posterior border. The diaphragm consists of the urethral sphincter sandwiched between two layers of fascia. The superficial perineal pouch is limited inferiorly by superficial fascia, the posterior edge of which is attached to the free posterior border of the urogenital diaphragm. The space thus formed is continuous with the scrotal sac and contains superficial perineal muscles and the root of the penis.

The anal triangle consists largely of the paired ischiorectal fossae, fat-filled spaces lying on either side of the anal canal (Fig. 3.4). These communicate with each other anteriorly by extending forward to occupy the deep perineal pouch of the urogenital triangle. The pudendal canal lies on the lateral wall of each ischiorectal fossa and transmits the pudendal nerve and internal pudendal vessels.

The anal canal, the terminal part of the alimentary tract, traverses the anal triangle in the midline. It is 4 cm long. Continence is maintained by the involuntary action of the internal sphincter, a condensation of circular muscularis fibres, and by the voluntary action of the external sphincter.

The penis is the erectile organ of copulation, comprising three masses of expansile tissue: the single ventral corpus spongiosum and the paired dorsal corpora cavernosa. The corpus spongiosum forms a cylinder around the penile urethra and is expanded at each end to form the glans penis anteriorly and the bulb of the penis posteriorly. The corpora cavernosa are joined in the midline for most of their length but diverge posteriorly to form the crura of the penis. The corpora are mostly subcutaneous except posteriorly where they lie in the superficial perineal pouch and are attached, by ligaments, to the pubic symphysis and the inferior layer of the urogenital diaphragm. They consist of fibrous envelopes divided into vascular spaces by trabeculae.

Vascular anatomy:

    arterial: branches of the internal pudendal arteries

    venous: tributaries of the internal pudendal veins

    lymph: superficial inguinal nodes

Methods of imaging the penis:

    radiographic: cavernosography

    ultrasonographic: real-time B-mode

THE MALE URETHRA

The male urethra is the common outlet of the urinary and reproductive systems. It is a curved muscular tube running from the internal urethral orifice in the bladder to the urethral meatus on the glans penis (Fig. 3.5). The posterior urethra is 4 cm long and pierces the prostate gland and the urogenital diaphragm. The anterior urethra is 16 cm long and lies within the corpus spongiosum of the penis.

   The lumen of the urethra is widest within the prostate gland and narrowest within the urogenital diaphragm. It is dilated anteriorly to form the navicular fossa in the glans penis and posteriorly to form the infrabulbar fossa in the root of the penis. Continence is maintained by the involuntary action of the vesical sphincter, part of the bladder muscularis, and by the voluntary action of the urethral sphincter, in the urogenital diaphragm. In the prostate gland the posterior wall of the urethra forms the urethral crest, a longitudinal fold, on to which the midline prostatic utricle and the two ejaculatory ducts open. Numerous prostatic ducts convey glandular secretions into the recesses on either side of the urethral crest. In the urogenital diaphragm two bulbourethral glands open into the urethral lumen.

Vascular anatomy:

   arterial: inferior vesical arteries
                internal pudendal arteries

   venous: prostatic plexus, draining into the internal iliac veins
                   and the internal vertebral plexus
                internal pudendal veins

   lymph: superficial inguinal nodes
                internal iliac nodes

Methods of imaging the male urethra:

   radiographic: ascending urethrography
                     micturating cystourethrography

   ultrasonographic: intrarectal micturating
                         endosonography

THE COMMON ILIAC ARTERIES

The common iliac arteries commence at the bifurcation of the aorta in front of the body of L4. They pass downward and laterally into the pelvis, where they are retroperitoneal, and divide into internal and external iliac arteries in front of the sacroiliac joints. The right common iliac artery is 5 cm long; the left is 4 cm long.

Relations of the right common iliac artery (Figs. 2.11, 3.2):

anterior:	small bowel
	ureter

posterior:	confluence of the iliac veins
	right common iliac vein
	sympathetic trunk
	lumbosacral trunk
	obturator nerve
	vertebral column

lateral:	psoas

Relations of the left common iliac artery:

anterior:	small bowel
	ureter
	root of the sigmoid mesentery
	superior rectal vessels

posterior:	left common iliac vein
	sympathetic trunk
	lumbosacral trunk
	obturator nerve
	vertebral column

lateral:	psoas

Methods of imaging the common iliac arteries:

radiographic:	femoral arteriography
	translumbar aortography
	computed tomography

ultrasonographic:	real-time B-mode
	Doppler

THE INTERNAL ILIAC ARTERIES

Each internal iliac artery commences at the bifurcation of the common iliac artery in front of the sacroiliac joint. It descends on the posterior pelvic wall and divides into anterior and posterior trunks (Fig. 3.6). It is 4 cm long.

The anterior trunk gives rise to branches supplying the pelvic viscera, the perineum and the hip joint and associated muscles. The umbilical artery, usually arising from the superior vesical artery, is obliterated after birth.

The posterior trunk gives rise to branches supplying the lower vertebral column and spinal cord, spinal muscles and gluteal muscles. *Methods of imaging the internal iliac arteries*: as for the common iliac arteries, p.97.

THE EXTERNAL ILIAC ARTERIES

Each external iliac artery commences at the bifurcation of the common iliac artery in front of the sacroiliac joint. It passes downward, forward and laterally on the pelvic wall and leaves the pelvic cavity through the femoral ring, below the inguinal ligament. At its origin it is anterior to the external iliac vein; at the femoral ring it is lateral to the vein. The vas deferens is medial to these vessels in its extraperitoneal course on the pelvic wall. The external iliac artery continues as the femoral artery below the inguinal ligament and gives rise to the inferior epigastric and circumflex iliac arteries.
Methods of imaging the external iliac arteries: as for the common iliac arteries, p.97.

THE ILIAC VEINS

The iliac veins and their tributaries correspond to the iliac arteries and their branches. Each external iliac vein lies medial to the artery at the femoral ring but becomes posterior as it ascends on the pelvic wall. The common iliac veins unite to become the inferior vena cava behind the right common iliac artery at the level of L5.

Methods of imaging the iliac veins:

radiographic: ascending iliac venography
                  computed tomography

ultrasonographic: real-time B-mode

In this chapter the organs of the female genital tract are described in detail. Structures common to both sexes are discussed briefly and the reader is referred to the corresponding section in Chapter 3.

THE SIGMOID COLON AND RECTUM

The sigmoid colon and rectum are similar in both sexes with the exception of the anterior relations. The peritoneum extends inferiorly in front of the rectum as the rectouterine pouch.

Relations of the female rectum:

      anterior: rectouterine pouch
                    bladder
                    cervix
                    vagina

THE BLADDER

The female bladder differs from that of the male in its inferior supports, its peritoneal covering and its relations.

As in the male pelvis, the bladder is suspended from the anterior abdominal wall by the median umbilical ligament. Inferior supports comprise condensations of pelvic fascia which are similar to those of the male except anteriorly, where paired pubovesical ligaments correspond to the puboprostatic ligaments.

The superior surface of the female bladder is covered by peritoneum on its anterior portion, the uterus overlying the remainder. The posterior peritoneal reflection therefore lies further forward than in the male and forms the uterovesical pouch.

Relations (Figs. 4.1, 4.2, 4.4):

      superior: small bowel
                   sigmoid colon
                   uterus

inferolateral: pubic bones
                   levator ani
                   obturator internus

posterior: cervix
             vagina

Vascular anatomy and methods of imaging: as for the male, p.83

THE UTERUS

The uterus is the female reproductive organ which provides a protective environment for the developing fetus and assists in its expulsion at parturition. It lies in the pelvic cavity between the bladder and the rectum. The non-pregnant uterus is a pear-shaped muscular sac consisting of a body and fundus anteriorly, with the cervix forming its posterior outlet. It is 8 cm long and 5 cm across. Each uterine tube arises from the junction between the fundus and the body of the uterus and extends laterally toward the pelvic wall and ovary. The upper vagina envelops the cervix, forming posterior and lateral fornices around it. The long axis of the uterus lies horizontally in the sagittal plane and at right angles to the vagina. When in this position the uterus is said to be anteverted. In transverse section the uterus is crescentic and its cavity forms a transverse slit.

The uterus is supported by paired round ligaments, each consisting of a fibromuscular band extending from the labium majorum, through the deep inguinal ring, to attach to the body of the uterus near the insertion of the uterine tube. This continues laterally as the ovarian ligament, which is connected to the corresponding ovary. Inferiorly the uterus is supported on levator ani by condensations of pelvic fascia around the cervix.

The uterus is covered by peritoneum on all but the inferior surface, where it is in direct contact with the bladder. The anterior reflection forms the uterovesical pouch. The posterior reflection forms the rectouterine pouch, a deep potential space between the upper vagina and rectum. The paired broad ligaments are folds of peritoneum which extend laterally to the pelvic wall, enveloping the uterine tubes, uterine vessels, ovarian ligament and round ligament.

The uterus is lined by endometrium, a vascular and secretory tissue which alters with the cyclical changes in circulating female hormones. The uterine cavity communicates, via the uterine tubes, with the peritoneal cavity and, via the internal and external os of the cervix, with the vagina.

Relations (Figs. 4.1, 4.2, 4.4):

    superior: small bowel
                  sigmoid colon

    inferior: bladder
                  vagina

    posterior: posterior fornix
                  rectouterine pouch
                  rectum

    lateral: broad ligaments
                  uterine tubes
                  ovaries
                  lateral fornices

Vascular anatomy:

    arterial: uterine arteries

    venous: uterine plexus, draining into the internal iliac veins

    lymph: external iliac nodes
                  para-aortic nodes

Methods of imaging the uterus:

    radiographic: plain films and tomography
                         computed tomography
                         hysterosalpingography

    ultrasonographic: real-time B-mode
                               endosonic

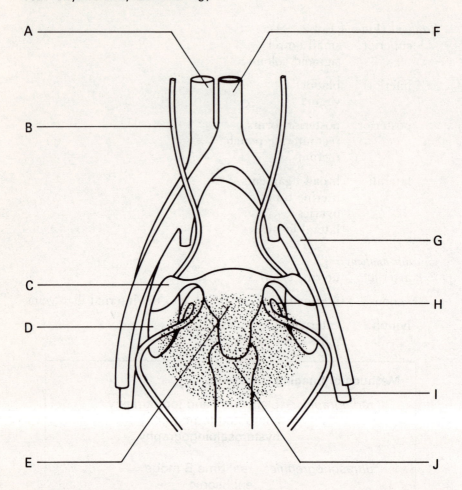

Fig. 4.1 *Structures behind the female bladder*

A: inferior vena cava
B: ureter
C: uterine tube
D: ovary
E: uterus

F: aorta
G: external iliac artery
H: ovarian ligament
I: round ligament
J: cervix

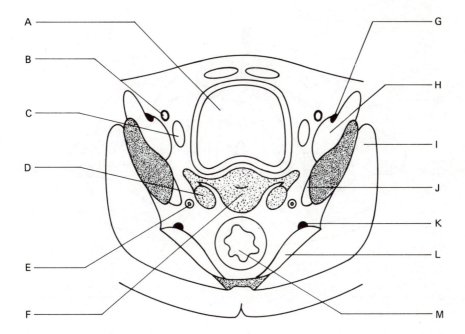

Fig. 4.2 *Cross section through the female pelvis at the level of the anterior inferior iliac spine*

A: bladder
B: femoral artery
C: femoral vein
D: ovary
E: ureter
F: uterus

G: femoral nerve
H: iliopsoas
I: gluteal muscles
J: obturator internus
K: sciatic nerve
L: piriformis
M: rectum

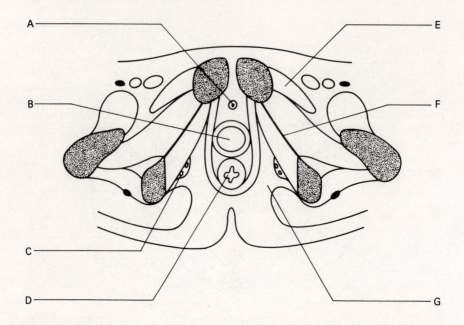

Fig. 4.3 *Cross section through the female pelvis at the level of the pubic symphysis*

A: urethra
B: vagina
C: pudendal canal
D: anal canal

E: pectineus
F: obturator membrane
G: ischiorectal fossa

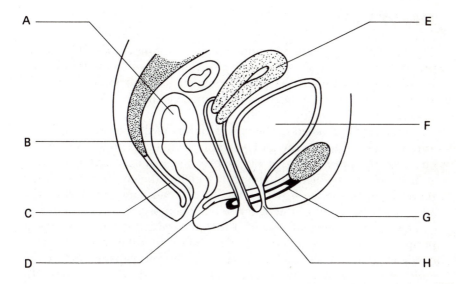

Fig. 4.4   *Sagittal section through the female pelvis*

A: rectum
B: vagina
C: levator ani
D: levator ani

E: uterus
F: bladder
G: urogenital diaphragm
H: urethra

THE UTERINE TUBES

These structures convey ova from the ovaries to the uterine cavity. Each extends from the junction of the body and the fundus of the uterus laterally to the ovary, over which it arches (Figs. 4.1, 4.2). It is 10 cm long. From medial to lateral it is divided into four segments: the uterine segment, isthmus, ampulla and infundibulum. The uterine segment has a lumen lying within the uterine wall; the isthmus is narrow and leads to the ampulla, which forms an expanded segment; the infundibulum forms a funnel-shaped opening into the peritoneal cavity and has finger-like fimbriae around its circumference which are closely related to the ovary.

Each uterine tube lies in the superior border of the broad ligament and is enveloped in peritoneum.

The lumen of the uterine part, isthmus and ampulla is narrow and lined by mucosa with numerous longitudinal folds.

Vascular anatomy and methods of imaging the uterine tubes: as for the uterus, p.101.

THE OVARIES

The ovaries are reproductive and endocrine organs responsible for the production of ova. They occupy a variable position in the pelvis. Each ovary is almond-shaped, having medial and lateral surfaces, anterior and posterior borders and superior and inferior poles. Its dimensions are 2 cm by 3 cm by 4 cm.

The ovary is attached to the infundibulum of the uterine tube by its anterior border and to the mesovarium, a fold of peritoneum continuous with the posterior layer of the broad ligament. Further support is provided by the ovarian ligament, which is the continuation of the round ligament between the layers of the broad ligament, and by the suspensory ligament of the ovary, a reflection of parietal peritoneum.

The ovary consists of a central medulla, which is vascular, and a peripheral cortex, which is cellular. The outer layer of cortex is condensed to form the tunica albuginea, a fibrous capsule. Before the endocrine menarche the ovary is smooth and homogeneous. In women of child-bearing age the cortex contains cyst-like follicles at different stages of development, corpora lutea and scarred areas corresponding to ruptured follicles. In postmenopausal women there is no further follicle development and the ovary is atrophic.

Relations (Figs. 4.1, 4.2):

anterior:	broad ligament
	external iliac vein
posterior:	ureter
	internal iliac vessels
superior:	uterine tube
inferior:	levator ani
medial:	uterus
lateral:	obturator vessels and nerve
	pelvic wall

Vascular anatomy (Fig. 2.11):

arterial:	ovarian artery, arising from the aorta
venous:	pampiniform plexus, draining into the inferior vena cava/left renal vein
lymph:	para-aortic nodes

Methods of imaging the ovary:

radiographic: computed tomography

ultrasonographic: real-time B-mode
                          endosonic

THE FEMALE PERINEUM, VULVA AND VAGINA

The female perineum, like that of the male, is divided into an anterior urogenital triangle and a posterior anal triangle, with the former divided into superficial and deep perineal pouches by the urogenital diaphragm.

The urogenital diaphragm is pierced by the vagina as well as the urethra (Fig. 4.4). The labia majora form the inferior limit of the superficial pouch and correspond to the scrotal sac.

The anal triangle and deep pouch of the urogenital triangle are very similar to those of the male. The erectile tissue and muscles of the female superficial pouch form the clitoris and vestibular bulbs, corresponding to the anterior and posterior parts of the penis, respectively. The vestibular bulbs lie on either side of the vestibule, into which the urethra and vagina open. They are covered by labia minora, folds of skin which lie medial to the labia majora. The labia, clitoris, vestibular bulbs and vestibule together comprise the vulva.

The vagina is a muscular tube lying between the bladder and the rectum in the midline (Figs. 4.3, 4.4). Its upper end envelops the cervix, forming lateral and posterior fornices, and it pierces the pelvic floor and urogenital diaphragm to open into the vestibule behind the urethra. It is 8 cm long.

THE FEMALE URETHRA

The female urethra extends from the internal urethral orifice of the bladder, piercing the pelvic floor and urogenital diaphragm to open into the vestibule between the clitoris and the vagina (Figs. 4.3, 4.4). It is 4 cm long.

5 | The Head and Neck

The cranial vault of the skull (Figs. 5.1, 5.2) consists of several bones connected by sutures, which are fibrous joints. The base of the skull consists of the sphenoid, occipital and paired temporal bones and is pierced by blood vessels, the spinal cord and cranial nerves. The facial bones provide a skeleton for the pharynx, nasal cavities, paranasal sinuses and eyes.

The vascular anatomy (Figs. 5.3–5.7) of the brain differs from that of non-nervous tissue by the presence of a 'blood–brain barrier', the absence of valves in the veins and the absence of lymphatic drainage.

The brain is normally demonstrated by plain films and tomography, computed tomography, arteriography and radionuclide scans. Ultrasonography may be used intraoperatively, in the presence of surgical defects and, via the fontanelles, in the newborn. Where relevant, the more specific investigations are listed.

THE BRAINSTEM

The brainstem serves as a conduit for nerves entering and leaving the brain and has important voluntary and involuntary functions. It lies in the posterior cranial fossa and consists of the medulla oblongata inferiorly and the pons and the midbrain superiorly (Figs. 5.10–5.12, 5.14, 5.15). The medulla is the continuation of the spinal cord above the foramen magnum and the midbrain consists of paired cerebral peduncles which connect the brainstem to the cerebrum and diencephalon. The pons is an anterior expansion between the medulla and the midbrain. The central spinal canal continues upward into the brainstem and is expanded to form the fourth ventricle, which communicates with the third ventricle, above, via the cerebral aqueduct.

The brainstem is traversed by all the nerve fibres entering and leaving the spinal cord. It contains the motor and sensory nuclei of the third to twelfth cranial nerves and the reticular formation, nuclei responsible for involuntary functions.

Vascular anatomy:

arterial:	vertebral arteries
	posterior cerebral arteries
venous:	basal veins
	great cerebral vein
	dural sinuses
	spinal veins

THE CEREBELLUM

The cerebellum coordinates voluntary and involuntary functions by modifying the motor output of the brain. It lies in the posterior cranial fossa behind the brainstem and consists of two hemispheres separated by the midline vermis (Figs. 5.9–5.12, 5.15). It has a superior surface, in contact with the tentorium cerebelli, and an inferior surface which is indented by the vallecula, a deep fissure in the midline. Each hemisphere is divided, by deep transverse fissures, into lobes and lobules, of which the tonsil is the most medial on the inferior surface. Shallower transverse grooves indent the cortex, forming folia. The cerebellum forms the roof of the fourth ventricle. It is connected to the brainstem by three pairs of cerebellar peduncles, which form most of the lateral boundaries of the fourth ventricle.

The cerebellum has a highly convoluted cortex of grey matter and several nuclei near the roof of the fourth ventricle. A branching network of white matter extends into it from the peduncles.

Vascular anatomy:

arterial:	superior cerebellar arteries
	anterior inferior cerebellar arteries
	posterior inferior cerebellar arteries
venous:	great cerebral vein
	dural sinuses

THE DIENCEPHALON

The diencephalon is the part of the forebrain that connects the cerebral hemispheres to each other and to the brainstem. It consists of those structures forming the walls, floor and roof of the third ventricle, which is the superior expansion of the cerebral aqueduct. The diencephalon lies in the middle cranial fossa (Figs. 5.8–5.10, 5.14, 5.15).

The thalami are paired groups of sensory nuclei which form most of the lateral walls of the third ventricle. Each is egg-shaped, with an anterior apex. They are usually connected, across the third ventricle, by the interthalamic adhesion. The medial and lateral geniculate bodies are two swellings on the posteroinferior surface of each thalamus.

The hypothalamus forms the lower lateral wall and the larger part of the floor of the third ventricle. It consists of the optic chiasm anteriorly, the paired mamillary bodies posteriorly and groups of autonomic nuclei above these. The tuber cinereum is an inferior swelling between the chiasm and the mamillary bodies and gives rise to the infundibulum of the pituitary gland. The posterior perforated substance and the subthalamic nuclei form the remainder of the floor of the third ventricle. The lamina terminalis forms the anterior wall and the habenular commissure, pineal body and posterior commissure form the posterior wall of the third ventricle. The roof is formed by a thin layer of ependyma.

Vascular anatomy:

arterial:	anterior cerebral arteries
	posterior cerebral arteries
	posterior communicating arteries
venous:	thalamostriate veins
	internal cerebral veins
portal:	hypophyseal portal veins, draining into the pituitary gland

THE CEREBRUM

The cerebrum, the major part of the forebrain, is the final destination of sensory input and the site of initiation of voluntary actions. It occupies the greater part of the cranial cavity, overlying the anterior fossa and the remainder of the brain (Figs. 5.8–5.12, 5.14). The two cerebral hemispheres are partly separated by the median longitudinal fissure. Each hemisphere has frontal, occipital and temporal poles and inferior, medial and lateral surfaces. It is divided into frontal, parietal, occipital and temporal lobes, each related to the corresponding bone of the cranial vault. The surface of the cerebrum is highly convoluted, with sulci forming indentations between gyri. The central sulcus separates the frontal and parietal lobes and the lateral sulcus (Sylvian fissure) separates these from the temporal lobe, overlying the insula, an invagination of the cerebral surface. There is no clear delineation of the occipital lobe. The paired lateral ventricles form the cavity of the cerebrum.

The cerebrum consists of an outer cortex of grey matter and contains the basal nuclei: the caudate and lentiform nuclei, the claustrum and the amygdaloid body. Sheets and bundles of white matter connect the cortex, nuclei and other parts of the brain: the internal capsule diverges from the cerebral peduncles into each hemisphere and continues, as the corona radiata, toward the cortex; the corpus callosum connects the hemispheres across the midline above the diencephalon; the optic radiation connects the optic chiasm to each occipital pole, running close to the inferior surface of each hemisphere. The olfactory nerves pierce the cribriform plate of the anterior fossa to enter the frontal lobes.

Vascular anatomy:

    arterial: anterior cerebral arteries
                   middle cerebral arteries
                   posterior cerebral arteries

    venous: superficial and deep cerebral veins

THE VENTRICLES

The ventricles are the cavities of the brain and are continuous with the spinal canal and the subarachnoid cisterns. They are lined by ependyma, which is invaginated in places by choroid plexus, a network of small blood vessels. Cerebrospinal fluid is secreted by the choroid plexus and circulates through the ventricles and spinal canal, draining into the cisterns via openings from the fourth ventricle (Fig. 5.15). The total volume of cerebrospinal fluid is 150 ml.

The fourth ventricle is the cavity of the brainstem. It is diamond-shaped when viewed from the front, having superolateral and infero-lateral walls formed by cerebellar peduncles. The rhomboid fossa is the floor of the fourth ventricle and is formed by the posterior surface of the pons and medulla. The roof is formed by the cerebellum and has a median dorsal recess and paired lateral dorsal recesses project-ing posteriorly into the cerebellum. Superiorly the fourth ventricle narrows to become the cerebral aqueduct and inferiorly it is continuous with the spinal canal. The median aperture of Magendie opens posteriorly, beneath the cerebellum, into the cisterna magna. Paired lateral recesses extend anteriorly between cerebellar peduncles to become the lateral apertures of Luschka, which open into the pontine cistern. Choroid plexus lines the roof of the fourth ventricle.

The third ventricle is a slit-like midline cavity in the diencephalon (Figs. 5.9, 5.10). It opens into the cerebral aqueduct inferiorly and communicates with the lateral ventricles anteriorly, via the interventricular foramina of Munro. The structures forming the walls, floor and roof are described above. The ventricle has optic and infundibular recesses in its floor anteriorly and a suprapineal recess at its posterior extremity. The ependymal roof separates the ventricle from the transverse fissure (Figs. 5.8, 5.15), from which paired longitudinal folds, containing choroid plexus, project downward.

The lateral ventricles (Figs. 5.8–5.10) are the cavities of the cerebral hemispheres. Each consists of a body with anterior, inferior and posterior horns in the shape of a 'C'. The anterior horns lie close to the midline, separated by the thin septum pellucidum. The bodies diverge posteriorly, separated by the splenium of the corpus callosum, and each follows the curve of the corresponding caudate nucleus, which forms most of the lateral wall of the ventricle. The third ventricle and the thalami lie in the concavity of the ventricles. Each inferior horn projects into the temporal lobe. Each posterior horn, though not always present, projects into the occipital lobe from the junction between the body and the inferior horn. Folds of ependyma, containing choroid plexus, project laterally from the tela choroidea of the third ventricle into the medial walls of the lateral ventricles, except in the posterior horns.

Vascular anatomy:

arterial:	choroidal branches of the internal carotid arteries
	choroidal branches of the posterior cerebral arteries
	posterior inferior cerebellar arteries
venous:	thalamostriate veins
	choroidal veins
	dural sinuses

Methods of imaging the ventricles:

radiographic: computed tomography
air ventriculography
contrast ventriculography

ultrasonographic: real-time B-mode

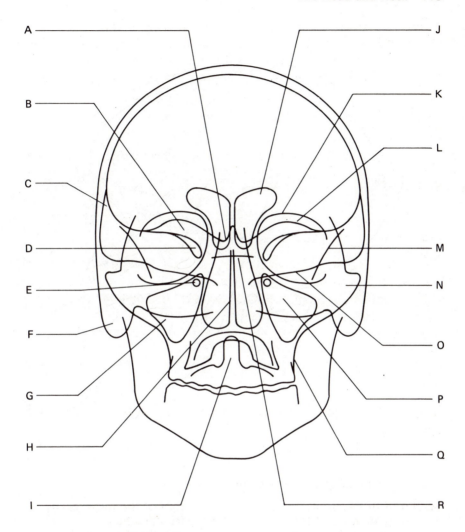

Fig. 5.1   *Frontal view of the skull*

A: roof of the nasal cavity
B: lesser wing of the
         sphenoid
C: greater wing of the
         sphenoid
D: superior orbital fissure
E: foramen rotundum
F: mastoid process
G: base of the skull
H: nasal septum
I: dens of the axis

J: frontal sinus
K: margin of the orbit
L: roof of the orbit
M: innominate line
N: zygomatic arch
O: petrous ridge
P: maxillary sinus
Q: superior alveolar process
R: floor of the pituitary fossa

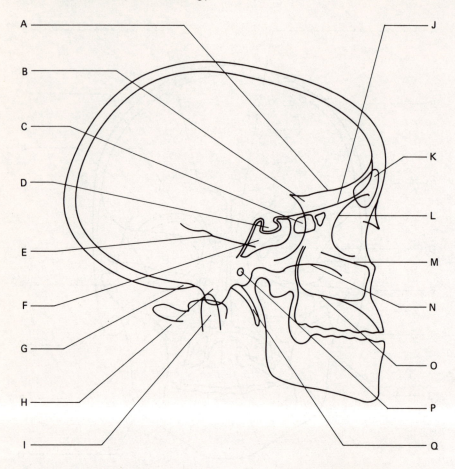

Fig. 5.2 *Lateral view of the skull*

A: roof of the orbit
B: greater wing of the
       sphenoid
C: ethmoid air cells
D: pituitary fossa
E: petrous ridge
F: sphenoid sinus
G: posterior margin of the
       foramen magnum
H: mastoid process
I: dens of the axis

J: roof of the nasal cavity
K: frontal sinus
L: margin of the orbit
M: floor of the orbit
N: inferior border of the
       zygomatic arch
O: hard palate
P: external auditory meatus
Q: styloid process

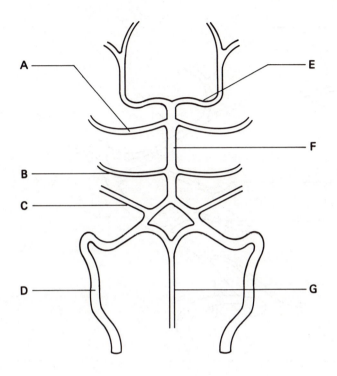

Fig. 5.3   *Frontal view of the vertebral arteries*

A: superior cerebellar artery
B: anterior inferior cerebellar
        artery
C: posterior inferior
        cerebellar artery
D: vertebral artery

E: posterior cerebral artery
F: basilar artery
G: anterior spinal artery

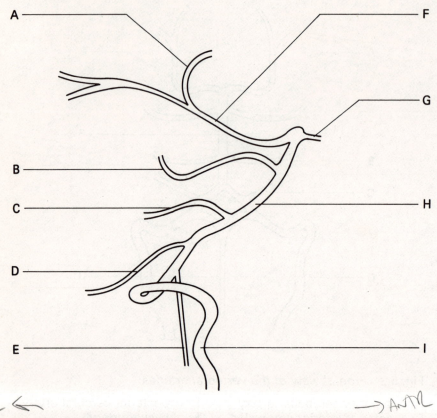

Posr ←   → ANTR

Fig 5.4 *Lateral view of the vertebral arteries*

A: posterior choroidal artery
B: superior cerebellar artery
C: anterior inferior cerebellar artery
D: posterior inferior cerebellar artery
E: anterior spinal artery

F: posterior cerebral artery
G: posterior communicating artery
H: basilar artery
I: vertebral artery

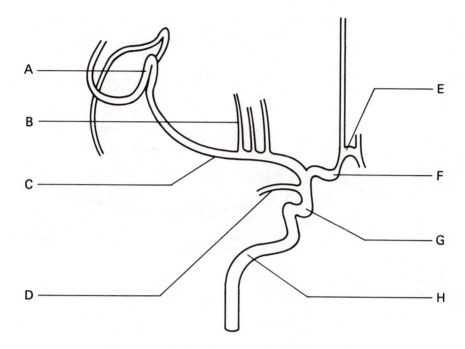

Fig. 5.5 *Frontal view of the right internal carotid artery*

A: insular course of middle
     cerebral artery
B: lenticulostriate arteries
C: middle cerebral artery
D: ophthalmic artery

E: anterior communicating
     artery
F: anterior cerebral artery
G: intracavernous part of the
     internal carotid artery
H: intrapetrous part of the
     internal carotid artery

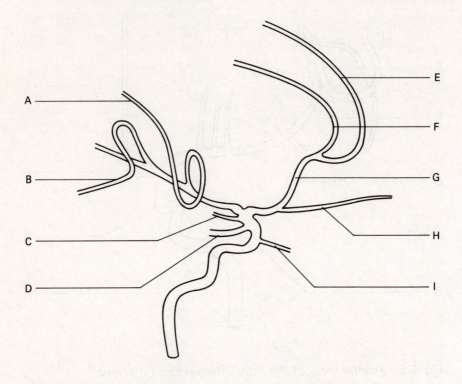

Fig. 5.6 *Lateral view of the internal carotid artery*

A: parietal branch of the
   middle cerebral artery
B: temporal branch of the
   middle cerebral artery
C: anterior choroidal artery
D: posterior communicating
   artery

E: callosomarginal artery
F: pericallosal artery
G: anterior cerebral artery
H: frontopolar artery
I: ophthalmic artery

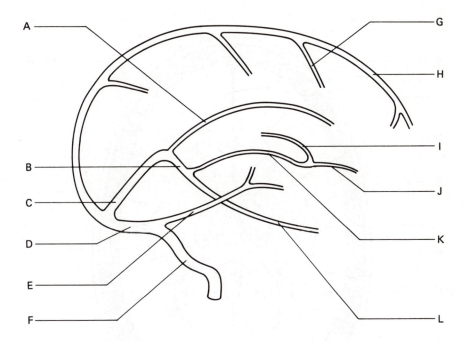

Fig. 5.7 *Lateral view of the venous drainage of the brain*

A: inferior sagittal sinus (unpaired)
B: great cerebral vein (unpaired)
C: straight sinus (unpaired)
D: transverse sinus
E: inferior anastomotic vein
F: sigmoid sinus

G: superior anastomatic vein
H: superior sagittal sinus (unpaired)
I: thalamostriate vein
J: septal vein
K: internal cerebral vein
L: basal vein

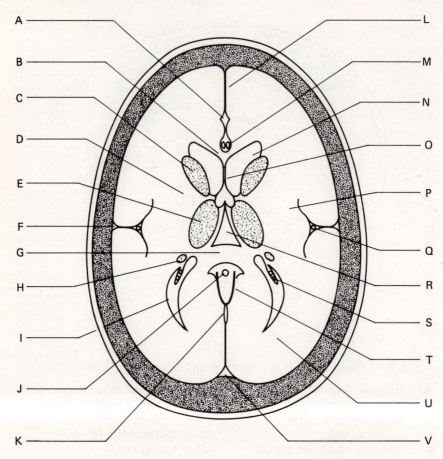

Fig. 5.8 *Cross section through the brain at the level of the transverse fissure* (JUST ABOVE III)

A: interhemispherical fissure
B: genu of the corpus callosum
C: head of the caudate nucleus
D: internal capsule/corona radiata
E: thalamus
F: central sulcus
G: splenium of the corpus callosum
H: tail of the caudate nucleus
I: posterior horn of the lateral ventricle
J: great cerebral vein
K: straight sinus
L: falx
M: anterior cerebral arteries
N: anterior horn of the lateral ventricle
O: septum pellucidum
P: insula
Q: middle cerebral artery
R: transverse fissure (ABOVE ROOF OF III ~ SUBARACHNOID SPACE)
S: choroid plexus
T: tentorium cerebelli
U: optic radiation
V: superior sagittal sinus

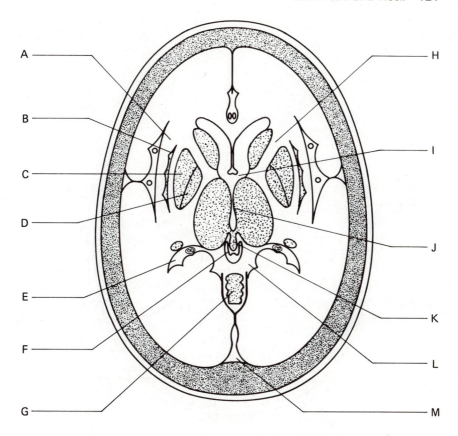

Fig. 5.9 *Cross section through the brain at the level of the interventricular foramina* (THRO ᗺ)

A: external capsule
B: claustrum
C: putamen of the lentiform
     nucleus
D: globus pallidus of the
     lentiform nucleus
E: temporal horn of the
     lateral ventricle
F: internal cerebral vein
G: vermis of the cerebellum

H: internal capsule
I: interventricular foramen (MonRoE)
J: third ventricle
K: pineal body
L: quadrigeminal cistern
M: confluence of sinuses

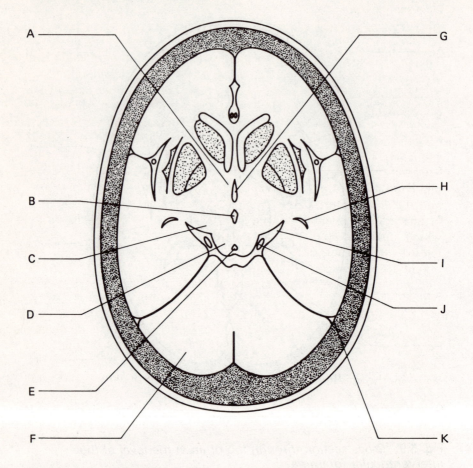

Fig. 5.10 *Cross section through the brain at the level of the floor of the third ventricle*

A: hypothalamus
B: interpenduncular cistern
C: cerebral peduncle
D: superior cerebellar peduncle
E: cerebral aqueduct
F: cerebellar hemisphere

G: third ventricle
H: temporal horn of the lateral ventricle
I: ambient cistern
J: posterior cerebral artery
K: sigmoid sinus

THE COVERINGS OF THE BRAIN

The brain is covered by three membranes. The pia mater is a thin layer of vascular and connective tissue which is closely adherent to the surface of the brain and the cranial nerves. It extends into the sulci of the cerebrum and into the fissures and grooves of the cerebellum. An invagination of pia mater forms the tela choroidea of the transverse fissure, between the roof of the third ventricle and the corpus callosum. This contains the internal cerebral veins and the vessels supplying the choroid plexus of the third and lateral ventricles. The tela choroidea of the fourth ventricle lies between its ependymal roof and the cerebellum.

The arachnoid mater is an avascular connective tissue membrane which surrounds the pia mater. Unlike the pia mater, however, it follows the internal contours of the skull. The subarachnoid space is a potential space between the arachnoid mater and pia mater. In places this is expanded to form the subarachnoid cisterns (Fig. 5.15), into which cerebrospinal fluid drains from the fourth ventricle.

The dura mater is the outermost covering of the brain, consisting of fibrous meningeal and endosteal layers. Reflections of the meningeal layer form folds which support the brain: the sickle-shaped falx cerebri extends from the crista galli to the internal occipital protuberance in the midline; the tentorium cerebelli is a tent-shaped fold covering the superior surface of the cerebellum, attached to the occipital bone and the petrous ridges; the diaphragma sellae roofs the pituitary fossa; the falx cerebelli extends from the internal occipital protuberance to the foramen magnum in the midline. Venous sinuses run between the two layers of the dura mater and arachnoid villi, projections of arachnoid mater through the meningeal layer, drain cerebrospinal fluid from the subarachnoid space into the dural venous sinuses. Groups of arachnoid villi are known as arachnoid granulations and are particularly prominent on either side of the sagittal suture.

Vascular anatomy:

arterial: ethmoidal, middle meningeal and occipital branches of the external carotid arteries
branches of the internal carotid arteries
branches of the vertebral arteries

venous: meningeal veins
dural sinuses

Methods of imaging the subarachnoid spaces:

radiographic: air encephalography
computed air or contrast
cisternography

radionuclide: ^{111}In-DTPA cistern scintigraphy

THE PITUITARY GLAND

The pituitary gland is an endocrine organ which lies in the pituitary fossa of the sphenoid bone, invaginating the diaphragma sellae. It has an ovoid shape, with an anteroposterior diameter of 8 mm and a transverse diameter of 12 mm. The gland is connected, by the infundibulum, to the tuber cinereum on the inferior surface of the hypothalamus (Fig. 5.15).

The gland consists of two parts: the posterior lobe and infundibulum are a downward extension of the floor of the third ventricle and have nerve connections with the hypothalamus; the anterior lobe secretes hormones in response to releasing factors conveyed from the hypothalamus by hypophyseal portal veins.

Relations:

anterior: sphenoid sinus

posterior: dorsum sellae of the sphenoid bone

superior: optic chiasm
hypothalamus
third ventricle

inferior: sphenoid bone

lateral: cavernous sinus

Vascular anatomy:

arterial: hypophyseal arteries, arising from the internal carotid arteries

portal: hypophyseal portal veins

venous: dural sinuses

THE CAVERNOUS SINUSES

The cavernous sinuses are paired dural venous sinuses which are connected to each other and to other veins and dural sinuses. They lie in the middle cranial fossa. Each is 2 cm long and 1 cm across.

Each sinus lies between the endostium lining the sphenoid bone and the meningeal layer of dura mater forming the diaphragma sellae. It is lined by trabeculated venous endothelium. The carotid siphon is the intracavernous portion of the internal carotid artery, traversing the floor and anterior wall of the cavernous sinus between the endostium and the venous endothelium. The third, fourth and sixth cranial nerves and the ophthalmic and maxillary divisions of the fifth cranial nerve also traverse the sinus.

Relations:

anterior:	orbit
posterior:	carotid canal
	apex of the petrous ridge
superior:	chiasmatic cistern
	optic nerve
	hypothalamus
inferior:	sphenoid bone
medial:	pituitary gland
	sphenoid sinus
lateral:	temporal lobes

Methods of imaging the cavernous sinus:

radiographic: computed tomography
orbital venography

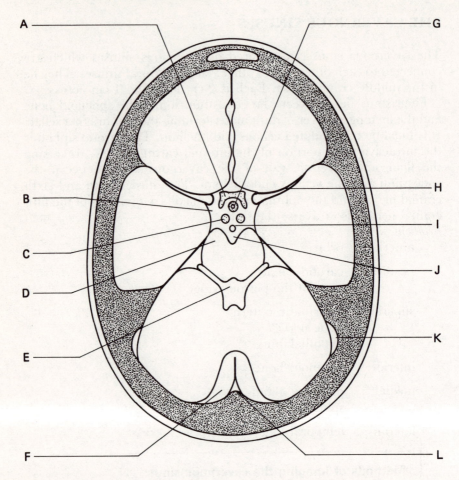

Fig. 5.11 *Cross section through the brain at the level of the chiasmatic cistern*

A: optic chiasm
B: chiasmatic cistern
C: mamillary body
D: cerebral peduncle
E: fourth ventricle
F: cisterna magna

G: infundibulum of the pituitary gland
H: middle cerebral artery
I: basilar artery
J: interpeduncular cistern
K: sigmoid sinus
L: occipital sinus

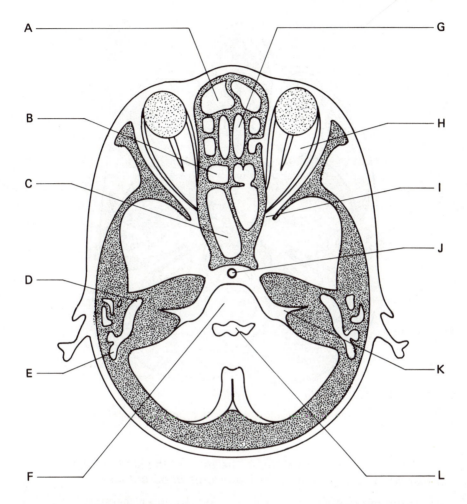

Fig. 5.12   *Cross section through the brain at the level of the pons*

A: frontal sinus
B: ethmoid sinus
C: sphenoid sinus
D: middle ear cavity
E: mastoid air cells
F: pons

G: nasal cavity
H: orbit
I: optic canal
J: basilar artery
K: internal auditory meatus
L: fourth ventricle

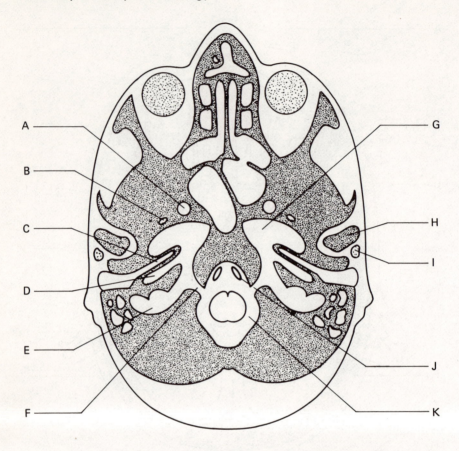

Fig. 5.13 *Cross section through the base of the skull (structures transmitted through the named apertures in parentheses)*

A: foramen ovale
       (mandibular division of
       the fifth nerve)
B: foramen spinosum
       (middle meningeal
       artery)
C: auditory tube
D: carotid canal (internal
       carotid artery)
E: jugular foramen (internal
       jugular vein, ninth,
       tenth and eleventh
       cranial nerves)
F: hypoglossal canal (twelfth)
       cranial nerve)

G: foramen lacerum
H: articular head of the
       mandible
I: parotid gland
J: vertebral artery
K: foramen magnum
       (medulla oblongata,
       vertebral arteries)

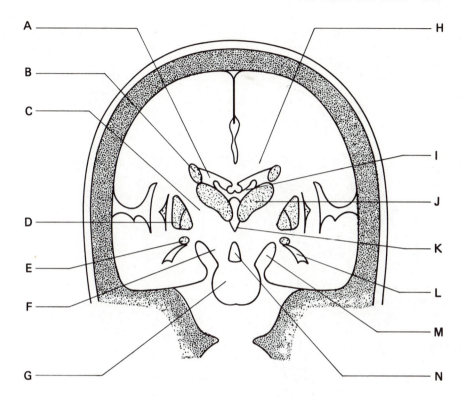

Fig. 5.14 *Coronal section through the brain at the level of the cerebral peduncles*

A: lateral ventricle
B: head of the caudate
        nucleus
C: internal capsule
D: lentiform nucleus
E: tail of the caudate
        nucleus
F: cerebral peduncle
G: pons

H: corpus callosum
I: transverse fissure
J: thalamus
K: third ventricle
L: temporal horn of the
        lateral ventricle
M: ambient cistern
N: interpeduncular cistern

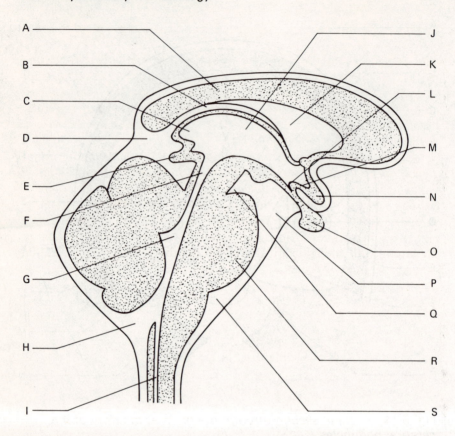

Fig. 5.15 *Sagittal section through the third ventricle*

A: corpus callosum
B: transverse fissure
C: suprapineal recess of the
       third ventricle
D: quadrigeminal cistern
E: pineal body
F: cerebral aqueduct
G: fourth ventricle
H: cisterna magna
I: spinal canal

J: third ventricle
K: septum pellucidum
L: infundibular recess of the
       third ventricle
M: optic recess of the third
       ventricle
N: optic chiasm
O: pituitary gland
P: chiasmatic cistern
Q: interpeduncular cistern
R: pons
S: pontine cistern

THE ORBITS

The orbits are cavities which contain and protect the eyes. Each is pyramidal in shape, having the optic canal at its apex. The roof, floor and walls are formed by the frontal, sphenoid, maxillary, lacrimal and ethmoid bones, the zygoma and the orbital process of the palatine bone. The orbit is limited anteriorly by the eye and by orbital fascia, covered by conjunctiva.

The optic canal transmits the optic nerve and ophthalmic artery. The superior orbital fissure (Fig. 5.1) separates the greater and lesser wings of the sphenoid bone and transmits the third, fourth and sixth cranial nerves, the ophthalmic division of the fifth cranial nerve, sympathetic nerves, the orbital branch of the middle meningeal artery and the ophthalmic veins. The inferior orbital fissure is an opening in the lateral wall and transmits the maxillary division of the fifth cranial nerve. The orbit also contains the bulbar muscles, the lacrimal gland and sac, and fat.

Relations (Figs. 5.12, 5.13, 5.17):

anterior:	palpebral fissure
	eyelid
posterior:	cavernous sinus
superior:	frontal sinus
	frontal lobe of the cerebrum
inferior:	maxillary sinus
medial:	ethmoid sinuses
	nasolacrimal duct
	nasal cavity
lateral:	temporalis muscle

Vascular anatomy: as for the eye, p.132, and lacrimal apparatus, p.134

THE EYES

The eyes are the organs of vision. Each lies in the anterior part of the orbit, embedded in orbital fascia and fat. The eye is approximately spherical and has an anterior pole and a posterior pole connected by the optical axis. At the anterior pole the sphere is distorted by the cornea, a transparent prominence. The eye is 22 mm in transverse diameter.

The eye has an outer fibrous sclera which is continuous with the cornea (Fig. 5.16). Within the sclera is the vascular uveal tract, consisting of the choroid, posteriorly, and the ciliary body and iris anteriorly. The ciliary body is a muscular ring surrounding and supporting the lens, whose shape it controls by contraction of radial or circumferential smooth muscle fibres. A similar arrangement in the iris, a thin diaphragm in front of the lens, controls the size of the pupil. The lens and its suspensory ligament separate the aqueous humour anteriorly from the vitreous humour posteriorly. The choroid is lined by the retina, whose most sensitive area, the macula, is at the posterior pole. The optic nerve leaves the eye at the optic disc, medial to the posterior pole.

The eye is enclosed in orbital fascia which is attached to the margin of the orbit, with thickenings forming the suspensory ligament below and the check ligaments on either side of the eye. Movement of the eye is controlled by rectus and oblique muscles attached to the circumference of the eye and to the walls and apex of the orbit.

Vascular anatomy:

      arterial: ophthalmic artery

      venous: ophthalmic veins, draining into the cavernous sinus

---

Methods of imaging the eye:

    radiographic: plain films and tomography
                    computed tomography

    ultrasonographic: real-time B-mode

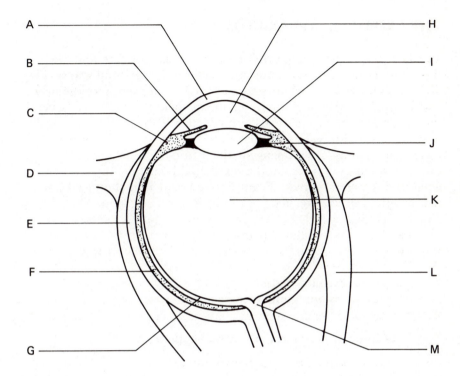

Fig. 5.16 *Transverse section through the eye*

A: cornea
B: iris
C: ciliary body
D: lateral check ligament
E: sclera
F: choroid
G: retina

H: aqueous humour
I: lens
J: suspensory ligament
K: vitreous humour
L: medial rectus muscle
M: optic nerve head

THE LACRIMAL APPARATUS

The lacrimal apparatus produces tears which lubricate and cleanse the conjunctiva. Secretions are produced by the lacrimal gland (Fig. 5.17), an almond-shaped structure at the lateral margin of the orbit, and drain into the upper part of the palpebral fissure via several ducts. Tears drain into two lacrimal canaliculi via puncta at the medial ends of the eyelids and pass into the lacrimal sac at the medial margin of the orbit. This opens inferiorly into the nasolacrimal duct, a canal between the maxilla and the lacrimal bone lined by epithelium whose folds act as valves. Tears finally drain into the nasal cavity beneath the inferior concha.

Vascular anatomy:

arterial:	ophthalmic artery
venous:	ophthalmic vein
lymph:	parotid nodes
	submandibular nodes

Methods of imaging the lacrimal apparatus:

radiographic: dacrocystography

radionuclide: ^{99m}Tc–colloid dacroscintigraphy

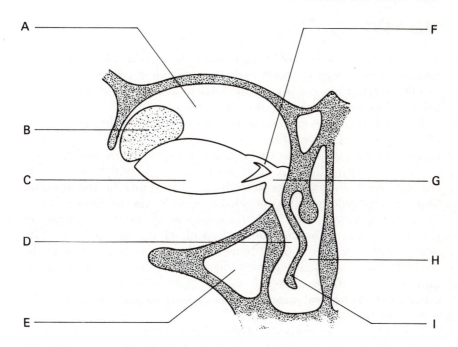

Fig. 5.17   *The lacrimal apparatus*

A: orbit
B: lacrimal gland
C: palpebral fissure
D: nasolacrimal duct
E: maxillary sinus

F: canaliculus
G: lacrimal sac
H: nasal cavity
I: inferior concha

THE EARS

The ears are the organs of hearing and balance. Each lies in a cavity formed by the temporal bone and the auricular cartilage.

The external ear consists of the auricle and the external acoustic meatus, limited medially by the tympanic membrane.

The middle ear is a narrow air-containing cavity in the petrous part of the temporal bone (Fig. 5.18). It lies between the tympanic membrane laterally and a thin layer of bone covering the structures of the internal ear medially. A superior expansion forms the epitympanic recess, which continues posteriorly as the aditus of the mastoid antrum. The middle ear is connected anteriorly, via the auditory tube, to the nasopharynx. The oval and round windows are openings, on the medial wall, into the bony labyrinth of the internal ear. The promontory is a projection of bone over the cochlea, anterior to the oval and round windows. The middle ear contains the malleus, incus and stapes, ossicles which conduct sound from the tympanic membrane to the oval window. It is crossed by the seventh cranial nerve and the chorda tympani.

The internal ear consists of fluid-filled membranous structures contained in the bony labyrinth, a cavity in the temporal bone medial to the middle ear. The bony labyrinth comprises the spiral cochlea and three semicircular canals, connected together by the vestibule, which communicates with the middle ear via the oval and round windows. It is lined by periosteum and contains perilymph, a fluid similar to cerebrospinal fluid, in which the membranous labyrinth is suspended. The membranous labyrinth comprises the saccule and utricle, the semicircular ducts and the cochlear duct, all of which contain endolymph, a fluid resembling intracellular fluid. Movement of, and vibration in, the fluids of the inner ear result in the perception of gravitational force, motion and sound waves. The auditory and vestibular divisions of the eighth cranial nerve pass medially from the internal ear to the posterior cranial fossa via the internal acoustic meatus.

Relations of the inner and middle ear (Fig.5.12):

superior:	temporal lobe of the cerebrum
inferior:	carotid artery
	jugular vein
	styloid process
anterior:	internal carotid artery
	auditory tube
	temporomandibular joint

posterior: mastoid air cells

posteromedial: brainstem
seventh and eighth cranial nerves
cerebellum
sigmoid sinus

Vascular anatomy:
arterial: branches of the internal carotid artery
maxillary artery
superficial temporal artery
labyrinthine artery, arising from the basilar or
anterior inferior cerebellar artery

venous: external jugular vein
dural sinuses

lymph: parotid nodes
retroauricular nodes
retropharyngeal nodes
superficial and deep cervical nodes

Methods of imaging the ear:

radiographic: plain films and tomography
computed tomography

THE NASAL CAVITIES

The paired nasal cavities form the uppermost part of the respiratory tract. They lie between the base of the skull and the hard palate. The roof, floor and lateral walls are formed by the nasal bones and cartilages, the maxillae, the inferior conchae and the frontal, ethmoid, sphenoid and palatine bones. The cavities are separated by the midline nasal septum, consisting of the vomer, the perpendicular plate of the ethmoid bone and the septal cartilage. Each nasal cavity is continuous with the vestibule of the nose, via the anterior nasal aperture, and with the nasopharynx, via the posterior nasal aperture, defined by the posterior border of the nasal septum. The superior and middle conchae are medial projections of the ethmoid bone into each cavity from the lateral wall. The inferior concha is a similar projection comprising a separate bone. The paranasal sinuses open into the nasal cavities via apertures on the lateral wall and the nasolacrimal ducts drain into the cavities beneath the inferior concha on each side.

The roof of the nasal cavities is lined by olfactory epithelium, supplied by branches of the olfactory nerve, which pierce the cribriform plate of the ethmoid bone. The remainder is lined by respiratory epithelium.

Relations (Figs. 5.12, 5.13, 5.17):

superior:	frontal lobe of the cerebrum
inferior:	oral cavity
anterior:	nose
posterior:	sphenoid sinus
	nasopharynx
lateral:	orbit
	nasolacrimal duct
	paranasal sinuses
	pterygopalatine fossa

Vascular anatomy:

arterial:	ophthalmic artery
	maxillary artery
	facial artery
venous:	ophthalmic vein
	maxillary vein
	facial vein
lymph:	submandibular nodes
	retropharyngeal nodes
	deep cervical nodes

Methods of imaging the nasal cavity:

radiographic: plain films and tomography
                  computed tomography

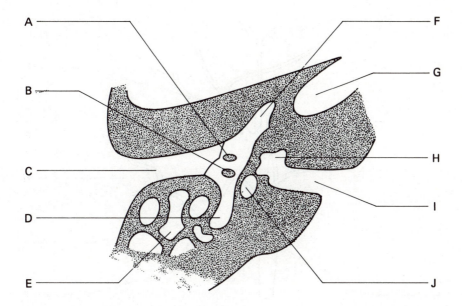

Fig. 5.18 *Cross section through the petrous temporal bone*

A: malleus
B: incus
C: external auditory meatus
D: aditus of the mastoid
     antrum
E: mastoid air cells

F: auditory tube
G: carotid canal
H: cochlea
I: internal auditory meatus
J: vestibule of the inner ear

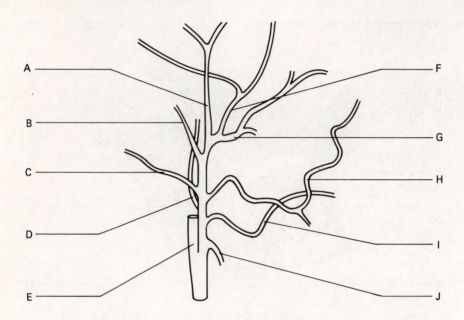

Fig. 5.19 *Lateral view of the external carotid artery*

A: superficial temporal artery
B: posterior auricular artery
C: occipital artery
D: ascending pharyngeal artery
E: internal carotid artery

F: middle meningeal artery
G: maxillary artery
H: facial artery
I: lingual artery
J: superior thyroid artery

THE PARANASAL SINUSES

The paranasal sinuses are irregular, air-containing cavities in the correspondingly-named bones which open into the nasal cavities (Figs. 5.12, 5.13, 5.17). The frontal sinuses are above the nose and orbits and in front of the anterior cranial fossa. The ethmoid sinsues lie between the upper nasal cavity medially and the orbit laterally. The sphenoid sinuses lie behind the upper part of the nasal cavities. The maxillary sinuses are lateral to the nasal cavities, below the orbits.

Vascular anatomy: as for the nasal cavity, p.138

Methods of imaging the paranasal sinuses:

radiographic: plain films and tomography
computed tomography

THE TEMPOROMANDIBULAR JOINTS

The temporomandibular joint is a synovial hinge joint between the condyle of the mandible and the mandibular fossa and articular tubercle of the temporal bone. Each joint is divided, by a fibrocartilaginous articular disc, into separate superior and inferior compartments (Fig. 5.20). The disc is attached to, and may be pulled forward by, the lateral pterygoid muscle. Rotational movement of the condyle of the mandible about a horizontal axis occurs in the inferior compartment. Forward movement of the condyle and the articular disc occurs in the superior compartment. These movements allow elevation and depression, protraction and retraction and lateral deviation of the mandible.

The joint capsule is attached around the neck of the mandible and to the articular margins of the temporal bone. A capsular thickening forms the lateral ligament, attached to the neck of the mandible and the zygomatic arch (Fig. 5.21).

The sphenomandibular ligament is attached to the sphenoid bone and the ramus of the mandible, medial to the joint. The stylomandibular ligament is attached to the styloid process and the posterior border of the ramus of the mandible, behind the joint.

Relations:

anterior:	lateral pterygoid muscle
posterior:	parotid gland external acoustic meatus
medial:	middle meningeal artery
lateral:	skin and fascia

Vascular anatomy:

arterial:	maxillary artery superficial temporal artery
venous:	maxillary vein superficial temporal vein
lymph:	parotid node deep cervical nodes

Methods of imaging the temporomandibular joint:

radiographic: plain films and tomography
computed tomography
arthrography

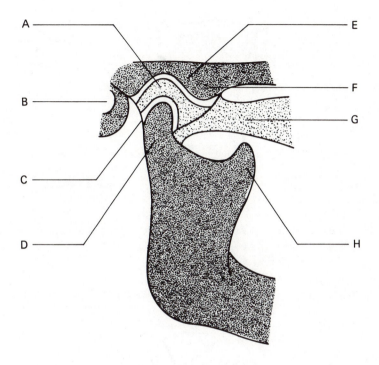

Fig. 5.20 *Parasagittal section through the temporomandibular joint*

A: articular disc
B: external acoustic meatus
C: joint capsule
D: condylar process of the mandible

E: mandibular fossa of the temporal bone
F: articular tubercle of the temporal bone
G: lateral pterygoid muscle
H: coronoid process of the mandible

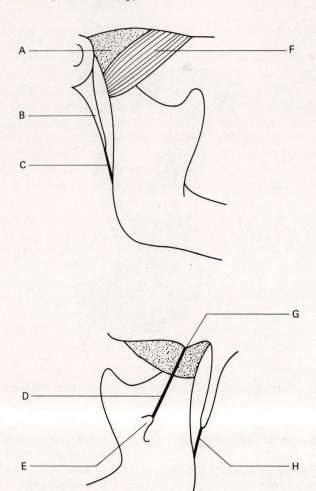

Fig. 5.21　*The temporomandibular joint*

A:　joint capsule
B:　styloid process
C:　stylomandibular ligament
D:　sphenomandibular
　　　ligament
E:　lingula of the mandible

F:　lateral ligament
G:　spine of the sphenoid
H:　stylomandibular ligament

THE PAROTID GLANDS

The parotid glands are exocrine organs responsible for the production of saliva. Each lies behind the posterior border of the ramus of the mandible, enveloped in cervical fascia. The parotid gland has an irregular shape with anteromedial, posteromedial and lateral surfaces, superior and inferior poles and anterior, posterior and medial borders. The parotid duct arises from the midpoint of the anterior border and runs forward to drain into the vestibule of the oral cavity, opposite the crown of the second upper molar tooth. The accessory parotid gland lies above the origin of the duct. The gland is 7 cm high and the duct is 5 cm long.

The parotid gland consists of serous secretory cells arranged in lobules, each drained by a single ductule. It is pierced by the external carotid artery and its terminal branches medially, by the retromandibular vein and by the seventh cranial nerve laterally.

Relations (Fig. 5.13):

anteromedial:	temporomandibular joint
	ramus of the mandible and attached muscles
	branches of the external carotid artery
	seventh cranial nerve
posteromedial:	external auditory meatus
	styloid process and attached muscles
	mastoid process
	sternocleidomastoid muscle
	external carotid artery
	seventh cranial nerve
lateral:	lymph nodes
	skin and fascia

Vascular anatomy:

arterial:	branches of the external carotid artery
venous:	external jugular vein
lymph:	parotid nodes
	deep cervical nodes

> **Methods of imaging the parotid gland:**
>
> *radiographic:*   plain films and tomography
>   sialography
>   computed tomography
>
> *ultrasonographic:*   real-time B-mode
>
> *radionuclide:* ^{99m}Tc-pertechnetate
>   sialoscintigraphy

THE SUBMANDIBULAR GLANDS

These salivary glands lie in the floor of the oral cavity, medial to the angle of the mandible. Each gland has an irregular shape and is divided into superficial and deep components by the mylohyoid muscle, which indents it anteriorly. The submandibular duct arises from the medial surface of the deep part of the gland and runs forward to open into the floor of the oral cavity. It is 5 cm long.

Vascular anatomy:

arterial:	facial artery
	lingual artery
venous:	facial vein
	lingual vein
lymph:	submandibular nodes
	deep cervical nodes

Methods of imaging the submandibular glands: as for the parotid gland, above.

THE SUBLINGUAL GLANDS

These paired salivary glands lie in the floor of the oral cavity, anterior to the submandibular glands and lateral to the submandibular ducts. Each has up to 20 ducts and the gland cannot therefore be demonstrated by sialography.

THE ORAL CAVITY

The oral cavity is the uppermost part of the alimentary tract. It extends from the lips to the anterior fauces and is continuous with the oropharynx posteriorly. The vestibule is the part of the oral cavity between the lips and the teeth. The parotid ducts open into the vestibule opposite the crowns of the second upper molar teeth; the submandibular and sublingual ducts open on to the floor of the oral cavity.

The tongue is a muscular projection from the floor of the mouth. It has an anterior tip and a convex upper surface which extends into the oropharynx. The anterior two thirds of the upper surface is covered by papillae. The tongue consists of intrinsic muscles attached to a midline fibrous septum and is connected, by extrinsic muscles, to the hyoid bone, palate and the styloid process of the temporal bone.

The soft palate (Fig. 5.24) is a muscular flap which closes the posterior nasal apertures during swallowing. It is attached to the posterior border of the hard palate and its paired muscular connections to the tongue and pharynx form the anterior and posterior fauces, respectively.

Teeth project from the alveolar processes of the maxilla and mandible. There are 20 deciduous and 32 permanent teeth. Each consists of a crown and a root composed of dentine (Fig. 5.22). The crown is covered by a layer of enamel and the root by a layer of cement. The root is attached to the lamina dura of its socket by the periodontal membrane, continuous with the periosteum of the alveolar process. It is traversed by the pulp canal, which contains blood vessels, nerves and connective tissue. The alveolar processes are covered by the gums, fibrous connective tissue and squamous epithelium, which form collars around the teeth.

Vascular anatomy:

arterial:	facial arteries
	maxillary arteries
	lingual arteries
venous:	facial veins
	maxillary veins
	lingual veins
lymph:	submandibular nodes
	submental nodes
	retropharyngeal nodes
	deep cervical nodes

Methods of imaging the oral cavity: as for the nasal cavity, p.138

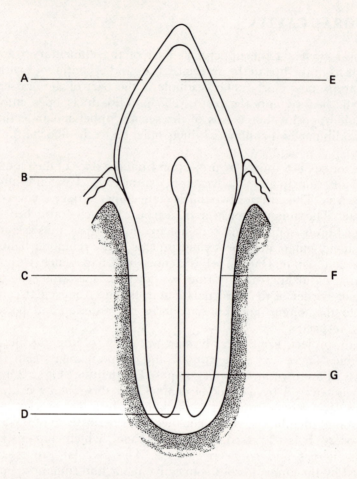

Fig. 5.22   *The structure of the tooth*

A: enamel
B: gingival epithelium
C: periodontal membrane
D: apical foramen

E: dentine
F: cement
G: pulp canal

THE PHARYNX

The pharynx is a muscular tube which is part of both the respiratory and alimentary tracts, connecting the nasal and oral cavities to the larynx and oesophagus. The greater part is in the neck, where it lies beneath the base of the skull and in front of the prevertebral fascia (Figs. 5.23, 5.24, 5.26). It is 14 cm long.

The nasopharynx is the backward continuation of the nasal cavities and extends from the posterior border of the nasal septum to the free border of the soft palate. It is roofed by the sphenoid and occipital bones and contains the adenoids, masses of submucosal lymphoid tissue on the posterior roof. The openings of the auditory tubes are on the lateral walls behind the inferior conchae.

The oropharynx is the backward continuation of the oral cavity and the downward continuation of the nasopharynx. It extends from the anterior fauces and the free border of the soft palate to the level of the upper border of the epiglottis. It contains the palatine tonsils, masses of submucosal lymphoid tissue between the anterior and posterior fauces on each side. The posterior third of the tongue forms its anterior wall.

The laryngopharynx is the downward continuation of the oropharynx. It opens into the oesophagus inferiorly, at the level of C6, and into the larynx anteriorly. The piriform fossae are paired recesses on either side of the laryngeal orifice, each lying between the aryepiglottic membrane medially and the lamina of the thyroid cartilage laterally.

The wall of the pharynx is formed by the superior, middle and inferior constrictor muscles. These are attached to a midline fibrous raphé posteriorly and to the sphenoid bone, the mandible, the hyoid bone and the cartilages of the larynx anteriorly. The nasopharynx is lined by respiratory epithelium and the remainder by squamous epithelium.

Vascular anatomy:

      arterial: maxillary arteries
                    facial arteries
                    lingual arteries
                    ascending pharyngeal arteries
                    superior thyroid arteries

      venous: pharyngeal plexus, draining into the jugular veins

      lymph: retropharyngeal nodes
                    deep cervical nodes

Methods of imaging the pharynx:

radiographic: plain films and tomography
barium swallow
computed tomography

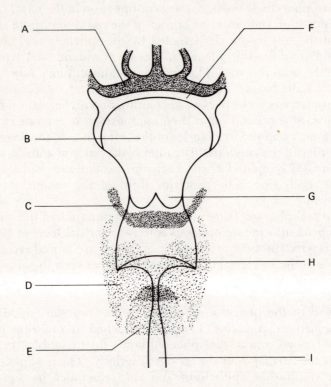

Fig. 5.23 *Frontal view of the pharynx*

A: hard palate
B tongue
C: hyoid bone
D: thyroid cartilage
E: cricoid cartilage

F: oral cavity
G: vallecula
H: piriform fossa
I: oesophagus

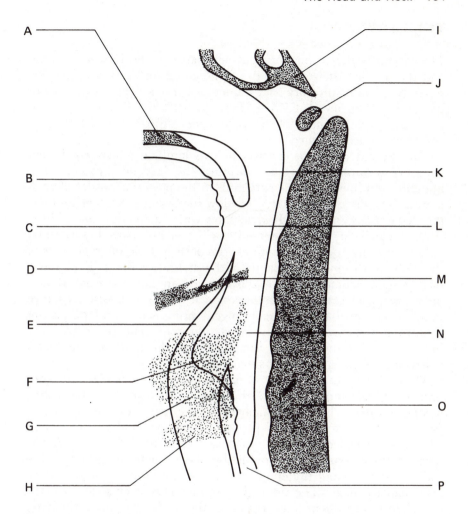

Fig. 5.24 *Lateral view of the pharynx*

A: hard palate
B: soft palate
C: tongue
D: vallecula
E: epiglottis
F: piriform fossa
G: thyroid cartilage
H: cricoid cartilage

I: sphenoid bone
J: anterior arch of the atlas
K: nasopharynx
L: oropharynx
M: hyoid bone
N: laryngopharynx
O: bodies of the cervical
        vertebrae
P: oesophagus

THE LARYNX

The larynx is the respiratory passage between the laryngopharynx and the trachea. It is the organ of phonation and serves as a valve separating the respiratory and alimentary tracts. The larynx lies in the neck at the level of C3–6 (Figs. 5.25, 5.26). It consists of an articulated cartilaginous skeleton to which fibroelastic membranes and muscles are attached.

The thyroid cartilage consists of two laminae which are joined along their anterior borders, forming the laryngeal prominence. Superior and inferior horns extend from the posterior border of each lamina. The cricoid cartilage lies below the thyroid cartilage and has the shape of a signet ring. It articulates with the inferior horns of the thyroid cartilage. The arytenoid cartilages are paired pyramidal structures lying above the posterior rim of the cricoid on either side of the midline, within the concavity of the thyroid cartilage. Each has a base, which articulates with the cricoid, an apex and vocal and muscular processes. The epiglottis is a leaf-shaped elastic structure attached to the back of the laryngeal prominence and projecting upward and backward into the laryngopharynx. The glossoepiglottic mucosal fold connects it to the tongue in the midline and forms valleculae, recesses on either side of the fold.

The conus elasticus consists of paired triangular elastic membranes attached to the superior rim of the cricoid cartilage. Each has a free medial border which is attached to the back of the laryngeal prominence and to the vocal process of an arytenoid cartilage, and which is thickened to form the vocal ligament. The aryepiglottic membranes are paired trapezoidal fibroelastic membranes attached to the lateral border of the epiglottis and to the anterior border of an arytenoid cartilage. The upper free border is thickened to form the aryepiglottic ligament and contains the triticeal and corniculate cartilages; the lower free border is thickened to form the vestibular ligament. The thyrohyoid membranes are paired fibrous structures which suspend the larynx from the hyoid bone.

The mucosa of the larynx is partly squamous and partly columnar epithelium. It is raised to form the vocal cords over the vocal ligament and the false cords over the vestibular ligament. The position of, and tension in, the vocal cords are adjusted by muscular action on the arytenoid cartilages. Movement of the larynx and apposition of the epiglottis over the laryngeal orifice isolate the respiratory tract from the alimentary tract during swallowing.

The rima glottidis is the midline aperture between the vocal cords. The sinuses are paired lateral recesses between the vocal cord and the false cord. The vestibule is the cavity above the false cords.

Relations:

superior:	fat-pad
	tongue
inferior:	trachea
anterior:	skin and fascia
anterolateral:	thyroid gland
	strap muscles
posterior:	pharynx

Vascular anatomy:

arterial:	superior thyroid arteries
	inferior thyroid arteries
venous:	superior thyroid veins
	middle thyroid veins
	inferior thyroid veins
lymph:	prelaryngeal nodes
	pretracheal nodes
	deep cervical nodes

Methods of imaging the larynx:

radiographic: plain films and tomography
computed tomography
laryngography

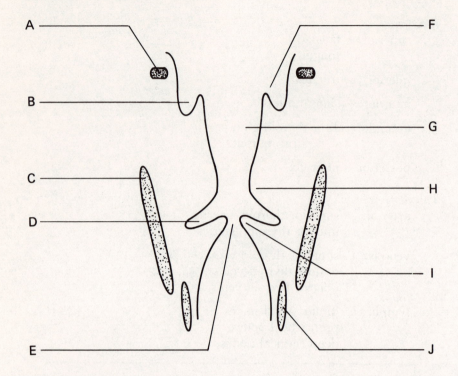

Fig. 5.25   *Coronal section through the larynx*

A: hyoid bone
B: vallecula
C: thyroid cartilage
D: sinus
E: rima glottidis

F: aryepiglottic fold
G: vestibule
H: false cord
I: vocal cord
J: cricoid cartilage

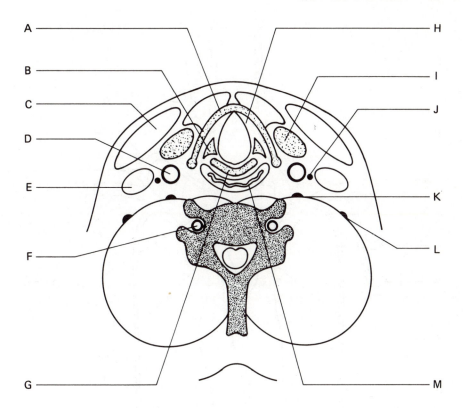

Fig. 5.26   *Cross section through the neck at the level of C6*

A: thyroid cartilage
B: arytenoid cartilage
C: sternocleidomastoid
D: common carotid artery
E: internal jugular vein
F: vertebral artery
G: cricoid cartilage

H: vocal cord
I: thyroid gland
J: vagus nerve
K: sympathetic chain
L: phrenic nerve
M: pharynx

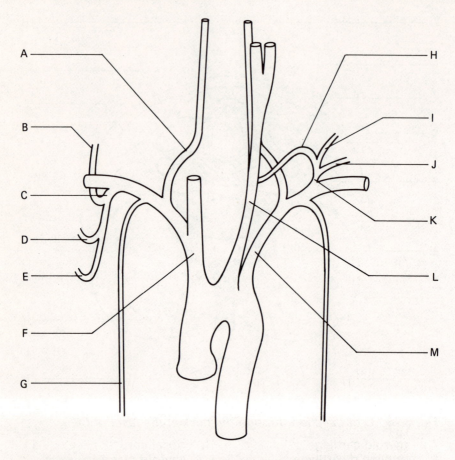

Fig. 5.27 *Arteries of the neck (for clarity some vessels are only shown on one side)*

A: vertebral artery
B: deep cervical artery
C: costocervical trunk
D: first posterior intercostal
      artery
E: second posterior
      intercostal artery
F: brachiocephalic artery
G: internal thoracic artery

H: inferior thyroid artery
I: transverse cervical artery
J: suprascapular artery
K: thyrocervical trunk
L: common carotid artery
M: subclavian artery

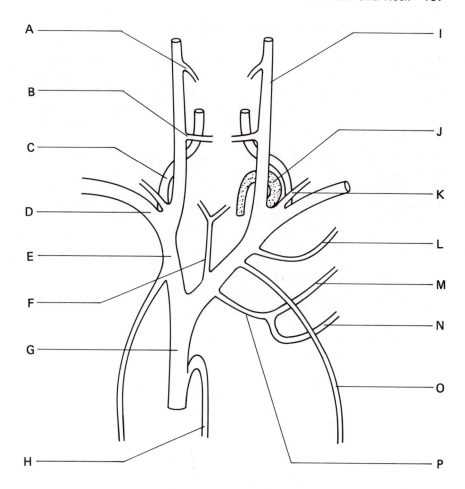

Fig. 5.28 *Veins of the neck*

A: superior thyroid vein
B: middle thyroid vein
C: vertebral vein
D: subclavian vein
E: brachiocephalic vein
F: inferior thyroid vein
G: superior vena cava
H: azygos vein

I: internal jugular vein
J: thoracic duct
K: external jugular vein
L: first posterior intercostal
    vein
M: second posterior
    intercostal vein
N: third posterior intercostal
    vein
O: internal thoracic vein
P: left superior intercostal
    vein

THE THYROID AND PARATHYROID GLANDS

The thyroid gland is responsible, under the influence of the pituitary gland, for the control of metabolic rate. It is enveloped in the pretracheal fascia of the neck and its two egg-shaped lobes lie on either side of the larynx and trachea at the level C5–T1 (Fig. 5.26). They are connected, in front of the trachea, by the isthmus. Each lobe is 5 cm high.

The four parathyroid glands secrete parathyroid hormone in response to serum calcium levels. They lie on the posterior surface of each thyroid lobe.

Relations of each thyroid lobe:

anterior: strap muscles
cervical fascia
sternocleidomastoid

posterior: parathyroid glands
thoracic duct (left lobe)
prevertebral fascia

medial: larynx
trachea
pharynx
oesophagus
recurrent laryngeal nerve

lateral: common carotid artery
internal jugular vein
vagus nerve

Vascular anatomy: as for the larynx, p.153

Methods of imaging the thyroid and parathyroid glands:

radiographic: plain films and tomography
computed tomography

ultrasonographic: real-time B-mode

radionuclide: ^{99m}Tc-pertechnetate thyroid
scintigraphy
radioiodine thyroid
scintigraphy
^{201}Tl thyroid and parathyroid
scintigraphy
^{99m}Tc(V)-DMSA medullary cell
scintigraphy

THE COMMON CAROTID ARTERIES

The right common carotid artery arises from the bifurcation of the brachiocephalic artery (Fig. 5.27). The left common carotid artery arises from the aortic arch and is partly in the neck and partly in the superior mediastinum. Both vessels ascend to the level of C4, where they divide into internal and external carotid arteries. The carotid sinus is a dilatation immediately below this bifurcation. Each artery is enveloped, with the corresponding internal jugular vein and vagus nerve, in the carotid sheath, a condensation of cervical fascia. The right common carotid artery is 10 cm long; the left is 12 cm long.

Relations of the left common carotid artery in the superior mediastinum (Fig. 1.7):

anterior:	manubrium
	left brachiocephalic vein
	thymus
posterior:	left subclavian artery
	left recurrent laryngeal nerve
right:	brachiocephalic artery
	trachea
left:	phrenic nerve
	vagus nerve
	left lung

Relations of the common carotid artery in the neck (Fig. 5.26):

anterolateral:	skin and fascia
	sternocleidomastoid
posterior:	sympathetic chain
	prevertebral fascia
	vertebral artery
	thoracic duct (left side)
medial:	larynx
	pharynx
	thyroid gland
	trachea
	oesophagus
	recurrent laryngeal nerve

lateral: internal jugular vein
              vagus nerve

Methods of imaging the common carotid artery:

radiographic: plain films and tomography
                  computed tomography
                  arch aortography

ultrasonographic: real-time B-mode
                      Doppler

THE INTERNAL CAROTID ARTERIES

Each internal carotid artery ascends from the level of C4 to the base of the skull (Fig. 5.27). It then follows a tortuous course through the carotid canal of the temporal bone and the cavernous sinus before dividing into its terminal branches in the chiasmatic cistern (Figs. 5.5, 5.6). There are no branches in the neck, where it is enveloped in the carotid sheath.

Relations in the neck:

medial:	pharynx
lateral:	styloid process and attached muscles external carotid artery internal jugular vein vagus nerve deep cervical lymph nodes sternocleidomastoid
posterior:	sympathetic chain prevertebral fascia

Relations in the skull:

medial:	sphenoid sinus
lateral:	middle ear auditory tube contents of the cavernous sinus anterior clinoid process
superior:	optic nerve

Methods of imaging the internal carotid artery:

radiographic:	plain films and tomography computed tomography carotid arteriography
ultrasonographic:	real-time B-mode Doppler

THE EXTERNAL CAROTID ARTERIES

Each external carotid artery ascends from the level of C4 to the parotid gland, in which it divides into the maxillary and superficial temporal arteries (Fig. 5.19). Branches supply the structures of the face and neck, the oral and nasal cavities and, via the middle meningeal artery, the meninges.

THE SUBCLAVIAN ARTERIES

The right subclavian artery arises from the brachiocephalic artery (Fig. 5.27). The left subclavian artery arises from the aortic arch and is partly in the neck and partly in the superior mediastinum. Each artery arches laterally over the apex of the lung, separated from it by the suprapleural membrane. It continues as the axillary artery at the outer border of the first rib.

THE INTERNAL JUGULAR VEINS

Each internal jugular vein is the extracranial continuation of the sigmoid sinus (Figs. 5.7, 5.28). It commences in the posterior part of the jugular foramen and descends to unite with the subclavian vein, forming the brachiocephalic vein. The internal jugular vein lies lateral to the common and internal carotid arteries in the carotid sheath (Fig. 5.26). It is 20 cm long.

Methods of imaging the internal jugular vein:

radiographic: plain films and tomography
computed tomography
retrograde internal jugular
venography

ultrasonographic: real-time B-mode

THE SUBCLAVIAN VEINS

Each subclavian vein is the continuation of the axillary vein medial to the outer border of the first rib (Fig. 5.28). It unites with the internal jugular vein to form the brachiocephalic vein. The vein is separated from the apex of the lung by the suprapleural membrane. It lies anterior to the subclavian artery, from which it is separated by the scalenus anterior muscle.

<table>
<tr><td>**6**</td><td>## The Spine</td></tr>
</table>

The spine consists of the vertebral bodies and the spinal cord. There are 33 vertebral bodies: seven cervical, 12 thoracic, five lumbar, five sacral and four coccygeal. The spinal cord gives rise to 31 pairs of segmental nerves: eight cervical, 12 thoracic, five lumbar, five sacral and one coccygeal. The first seven cervical nerves emerge above the correspondingly – numbered vertebral body; the remainder emerge below.

THE SPINAL CORD

The spinal cord is the downward continuation of the medulla in the vertebral canal. It extends from the foramen magnum to the conus medullaris at the level of the L1/2 disc and is 45 cm long It is cylindrical, with cervical and lumbar enlargements corresponding to the nerve roots supplying the upper and lower limbs. The cord is indented by the posteromedial, posterolateral and anterolateral sulci and by the deeper anteromedial fissure. The ventral nerve roots, containing motor and autonomic neurones, arise from the anterolateral sulci; the dorsal nerve roots, containing sensory neurones and ganglia, enter the cord in the posterolateral sulci. Ventral and dorsal nerve roots unite in intervertebral foramina to form segmental nerves. The lumbar and sacral nerve roots and the filum terminale, a fibrous band in the midline, form the cauda equina, which occupies the subarachnoid space below the conus medullaris. The central spinal canal runs the length of the cord and is continuous with the fourth ventricle of the brainstem.

The spinal cord and nerve roots are covered by pia mater, a vascular connective tissue continuous with that covering the brain. The cord is supported in the vertebral canal by the denticulate ligaments, sheets of pia mater attached to each side of the cord and, at intervals, to the dura mater lining the vertebral canal (Fig. 6.1) The subarachnoid septum is a perforated sheet of pia mater attached to the posterior median sulcus of the cord and to the dura mater of the vertebral canal in the midline. The arachnoid mater forms a sub-arachnoid space which is continuous with the cisterna magna and extends down to the level of S2. The dura mater lines the vertebral canal.

In transverse section the spinal cord has peripheral areas of white matter and a central area of grey matter. The reticular formation and some cranial nerve nuclei extend into the upper cord.

Vascular anatomy:

arterial: anterior spinal artery, a single midline artery arising from both vertebral arteries (Figs. 5.3, 5.4)

posterior spinal arteries, arising from the posterior inferior cerebellar arteries

*anterior radicular arteries ⎫ arising from the
posterior radicular arteries ⎭ segmental arteries

venous: anterior spinal veins
posterior spinal veins

Methods of imaging the spinal cord and canal:

radiographic: plain films and tomography
computed tomography
myelography
arteriography
ascending lumbar venography

ultrasonographic: real-time B-mode, through bony defects

radionuclide: ^{111}In-DTPA cistern scintigraphy

---

*The arteria radicularis magna of Adamkiewicz, a single enlarged anterior radicular artery, may supply a large proportion of the cord by anastomosing with the anterior and posterior spinal arteries.

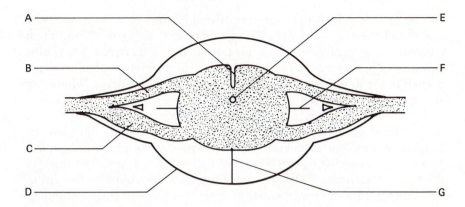

Fig 6.1 *Cross section through the spinal cord*

A: anterior median fissure
B: ventral nerve root
C: dorsal nerve root
    ganglion
D: dura mater

E: spinal canal
F: denticulate ligament
G: subarachnoid septum

THE VERTEBRAL COLUMN

The vertebral column supports the head, upper limbs and trunk on the pelvis, provides attachment for skeletal musculature and forms the protective vertebral canal for the spinal cord. It is 'S'-shaped, having cervical and lumbar lordoses and a thoracic kyphosis. It is 70 cm long.

Each vertebra consists of a cylindrical body anteriorly and a vertebral arch posteriorly (Figs. 6.2–6.6). The arch consists of paired pedicles and laminae and surrounds the vertebral foramen. The midline spinous process and paired transverse, superior articular and inferior articular processes are attached to the arch. Each articular process bears an articular facet. Each pedicle has superior and inferior vertebral notches which form the intervertebral foramina.

The vertebrae become progressively larger toward the pelvis. The vertebral foramina together form the vertebral canal, which is circular in the thoracic region but triangular in the cervical and lumbar regions. Cervical vertebrae have several distinctive features: the transverse processes are each pierced by a foramen transversarium; the atlas and axis (C1 and C2) are modified to allow movement of the skull on the cervical spine and the spinous processes of C2–6 are bifid. Thoracic vertebrae have costal facets, on the bodies and transverse processes, for articulation with ribs.

The intervertebral discs are fibrocartilaginous structures between the vertebral bodies which allow movement between them. Each consists of a central nucleus pulposus and a peripheral annulus fibrosus. The vertebral bodies and the intervertebral discs are attached to the anterior and posterior longitudinal ligaments, which run the length of the vertebral column.

The vertebral arches articulate with each other at the synovial facet joints. The ligamenta flava are paired elastic ligaments between the lamina of adjacent vertebrae. The intertransverse and interspinous ligaments connect the transverse and spinous processes, respectively, of adjacent vertebrae. The supraspinous ligament connects the tips of the spinous processes and runs the length of the vertebral column.

Vascular anatomy:

    arterial: vertebral arteries
                    ascending cervical arteries
                    intercostal arteries
                    lumbar arteries
                    lateral sacral arteries

    venous: vertebral plexuses, draining into the dural sinuses and vertebral, azygos, lumbar and internal iliac veins

    lymph: deep cervical nodes
                    intercostal nodes
                    para-aortic nodes
                    internal iliac nodes

Methods of imaging the vertebral column:

    radiographic: plain films and tomography
                          computed tomography
                          myelography
                          ascending lumbar venography
                          facet arthrography
                          discography

    radionuclide: ^{99m}Tc-diphosphonate bone scintigraphy

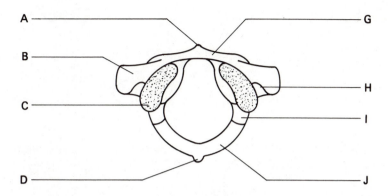

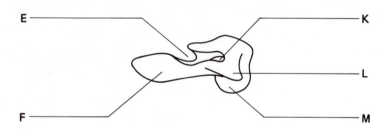

Fig. 6.2   *The atlas*

A: anterior tubercle
B: transverse process
C: superior articular facet of
    the lateral mass
D: posterior tubercle
E: groove for the vertebral
    artery
F: posterior arch

G: anterior arch
H: foramen transversarium
I: groove for the vertebral
    artery
J: posterior arch
K: foramen transversarium
L: transverse process
M: lateral mass

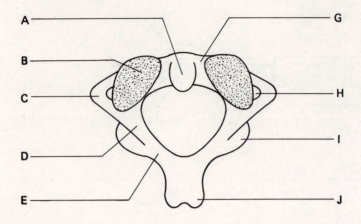

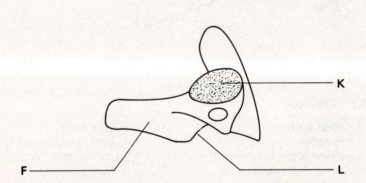

Fig. 6.3 *The axis*

A: dens
B: superior articular facet
C: transverse process
D: pedicle
E: lamina
F: spinous process

G: body
H: foramen transversarium
I: inferior articular process
J: spinous processes
K: superior articular facet
L: inferior articular process

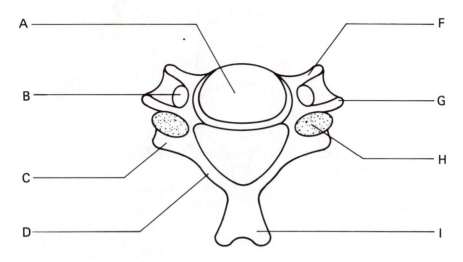

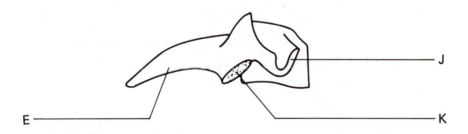

Fig. 6.4 *A typical cervical vertebra*

A: body
B: foramen transversarium
C: inferior articular process
D: lamina
E: spinous processes

F: anterior tubercle of the
   transverse process
G: posterior tubercle of the
   transverse process
H: superior articular facet
I: spinous processes
J: transverse process
K: inferior articular facet

AP obliques shows foramina furthest from film

Joints of Luschka C3-C7 inclusive

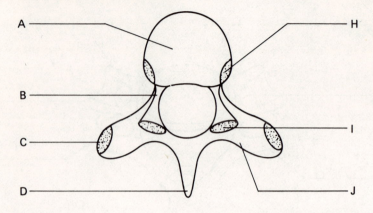

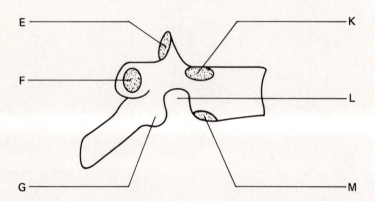

Fig. 6.5 *A typical thoracic vertebra*

A: body
B: lamina
C: costal facet
D: spinous process
E: superior articular facet
F: costal facet
G: inferior articular process

H: costal facet
I: superior articular facet
J: transverse process
K: costal facet
L: inferior notch
M: costal facet

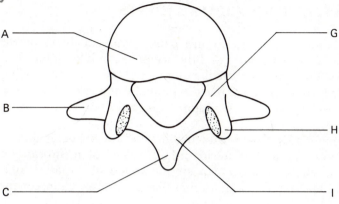

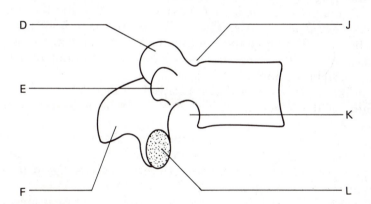

Fig. 6.6 *A typical lumbar vertebra*

A:	body	G:	pedicle
B:	transverse process	H:	superior articular process
C:	spinous process	I:	lamina
D:	superior articular process	J:	superior notch
E:	transverse process	K:	inferior notch
F:	spinous process	L:	inferior articular facet

AP oblique shows pedicles and foramina nearest film

THE ATLANTO-OCCIPITAL JOINTS

The atlanto-occipital joints are paired synovial joints between the superior facets of the atlas and the occipital condyles of the skull (Figs. 6.7, 6.8). The concave articular surfaces of the atlas face medially and are kidney-shaped. Together the joints form a condyloid joint which allows flexion, extension and limited lateral flexion of the head on the atlas.

The joint capsules are attached around the articular margins.

The anterior and posterior atlanto-occipital membranes are attached to the anterior and posterior arches of the atlas and to the occiput. The anterior longitudinal ligament also reinforces the joint.

THE ATLANTOAXIAL JOINTS

The three atlantoaxial joints are synovial joints between the atlas and the axis (Figs. 6.7, 6.8). The paired lateral atlantoaxial joints are plane joints between the lateral masses of the atlas and the superior articular facets of the axis. The median atlantoaxial joint is a pivot joint between the dens of the axis and the anterior arch and transverse ligament of the atlas. Together these joints allow rotation of the head on the vertebral column.

The lateral joints each have a capsule attached to the articular margins of the facets. Each is reinforced by an accessory ligament medially.

The median joint is divided, by the dens, into an anterior compartment where the dens articulates with the anterior arch and a posterior compartment where it articulates with the transverse ligament. Each compartment has a separate capsule.

The apical ligament is attached to the apex of the dens and to the occipital bone. The cruciate ligament consists of the transverse ligament, attached to the medial surface of each lateral mass of the atlas, and longitudinal bands attached to the occiput and the axis. The membrana tectoria is the continuation of the posterior longitudinal ligament. The paired alar ligaments are attached to the dens and the occipital condyles.

THE SACROILIAC JOINTS

The sacroiliac joint is a synovial plane joint between the auricular surface of the lateral part of the sacrum and the ilium (Fig. 3.1). Rotation occurs at each joint, allowing flexion of the spine on the pelvis. The range of movement is small and diminishes with age but during pregnancy the joint becomes more lax.

The joint capsule is attached to the articular margins. The interosseous sacroiliac ligament is a massive capsular thickening above and behind the articular surfaces. The ventral sacroiliac ligament is a anterior capsular thickening and the dorsal sacroiliac ligament is a posterior capsular thickening, behind the interosseous sacroiliac ligament.

The sacrotuberous ligament is an accessory ligament connecting the posterior surfaces of the sacrum and coccyx to the posterior iliac spines and the ischial tuberosity. The sacrospinous ligament connects the lateral border of the sacrum to the ischial spine, in front of the sacrotuberous ligament. The iliolumbar ligament connects the iliac crest to the transverse process of L5.

Relations:

anterior: lumbosacral nerve trunk
             obturator nerve
             psoas
             bifurcation of the common iliac artery
             confluence of the iliac veins
             ureter

Vascular anatomy: as for the vertebral column, p.168

Methods of imaging the sacroiliac joint:

radiographic: plain films and tomography
                  computed tomography
                  arthrography

radionuclide: ^{99m}Tc-diphosphonate bone
                  scintigraphy

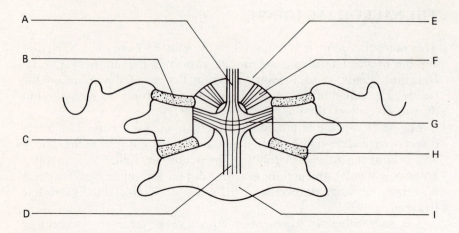

Fig. 6.7 *Posterior view of the atlanto-occipital and atlantoaxial joints (membrana tectoria not shown)*

A: superior longitudinal band of the cruciate ligament
B: atlanto-occipital joint
C: lateral mass of the atlas
D: inferior longitudinal band of the cruciate ligament

E: anterior margin of the foramen magnum
F: alar ligament
G: transverse band of the cruciate ligament
H: lateral atlantoaxial joint capsule
I: body of the axis

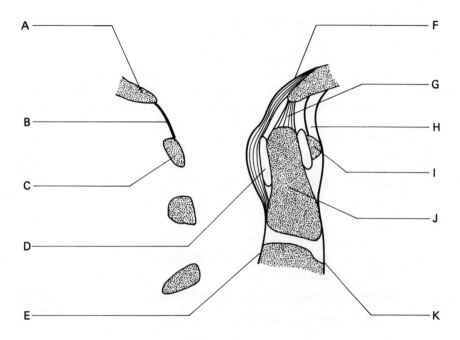

Fig. 6.8 *Sagittal section through the atlanto-occipital and atlantoaxial joints*

A: posterior margin of the
    foramen magnum
B: posterior atlanto-occipital
    membrane
C: posterior arch of the atlas
D: cruciate ligament
E: posterior longitudinal
    ligament

F: membrana tectoria
G: apical ligament of the
    dens
H: anterior atlanto-occipital
    membrane
I: anterior arch of the atlas
J: dens
K: anterior longitudinal
    ligament

LIGS. OF. DENS { ALAR(2) → ANTR FORAMEN MAGNUM
                  APICAL ↗ ⊥
                  CRUCIATE → ATLAS(2) ⊨
                    ⤹
                  FORMS JOINT
                  WITH DENS   BODY OF AXIS

THE VERTEBRAL ARTERIES

Each vertebral artery arises from the subclavian artery and ascends through the foramina transversaria of the upper six cervical vertebrae (Figs. 5.3, 5.4, 5.27). Above the posterior arch of the atlas it turns medially, piercing the posterior atlanto-occipital membrane, and then upward to enter the skull through the foramen magnum. The paired vertebral arteries unite to form the basilar artery in front of the brainstem.

Relations in the root of the neck:

      anterior: common carotid artery
                       thoracic duct (left side)

      posterior: prevertebral fascia
                       sympathetic chain
                       ventral roots of cervical nerves

Methods of imaging the vertebral artery:

   radiographic: plain films and tomography
                          computed tomography
                          arch aortography
                          vertebral arteriography

---

7 | The Upper Limb

The upper limb consists of the hand, forearm, arm and the structures comprising the shoulder girdle. The hand is used for manipulation and grip and the remainder of the upper limb is used to position the hand. Compared with the lower limb the joints allow a wider range of movement but are less stable; the muscles enhance fine control of movement at the expense of power.

THE SHOULDER JOINTS

The shoulder joint is a synovial ball-and-socket joint between the concave glenoid fossa of the scapula and the hemispherical head of the humerus. The relatively small area of the glenoid fossa and the laxity of the joint capsule accommodate a wide range of movement.

The joint capsule is attached around the circumference of the glenoid fossa, extending proximally to include the root of the coracoid process and distally on to the anatomical neck of the humerus. The capsule communicates with the subscapularis bursa, which lies anterior to the joint. The glenoid labrum forms a fibrocartilaginous rim to the glenoid fossa, increasing the area of its articular surface. The long head of biceps traverses the joint to attach to the base of the coracoid process above the glenoid fossa (Fig. 7.1). The synovial membrane of the joint forms a tubular sheath around the long head of biceps and is continuous with the synovial membrane lining the subscapularis bursa. The glenohumeral ligaments are three thickenings of the joint capsule which form anterior, reinforcements (Fig. 7.2).

The coracohumeral ligament is an accessory ligament attached to the base of the coracoid process and to the greater tuberosity of the humerus. The transverse humeral ligament is attached to the greater and lesser tuberosities, forming a tunnel for the long head of biceps. The coracoacromial ligament reinforces the joint superiorly.

Relations:

anterior: subscapularis bursa (COMMUNICATES WITH JOIN)
            rotator cuff muscles

posterior: rotator cuff muscles

superior: subacromial bursa (DOES NOT COMMUNICATE)
            rotator cuff muscles

inferior: long head of triceps
            axillary nerve

Vascular anatomy:

arterial: branches of the axillary artery

venous: venae comitantes, corresponding to arteries

lymph: axillary nodes
            deep cervical nodes

Methods of imaging the shoulder joint:

radiographic: plain films and tomography
                  computed tomography
                  arthrography (SC/DC)

radionuclide: ^{99m}Tc-diphosphonate bone
                  scintigraphy

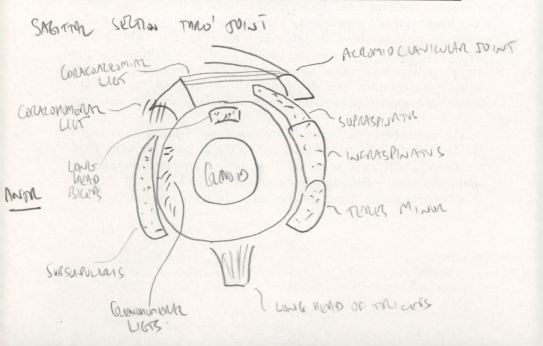

SAGITTAL SECTION THRO' JOINT

ACROMIOCLAVICULAR JOINT

CORACOACROMIAL LIGT

CORACOHUMERAL LIGT

LONG HEAD BICEPS

ANTR

GLENOID

SUPRASPINATUS

INFRASPINATUS

TERES MINOR

SUBSCAPULARIS

GLENOHUMERAL LIGTS

LONG HEAD OF TRICEPS

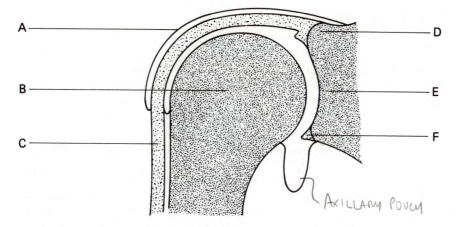

Fig. 7.1 *Coronal section through the shoulder joint*

A: joint capsule
B: head of the humerus
C: tendon of the long head
     of biceps

D: insertion of the long head
     of biceps
E: glenoid fossa
F: glenoid labrum

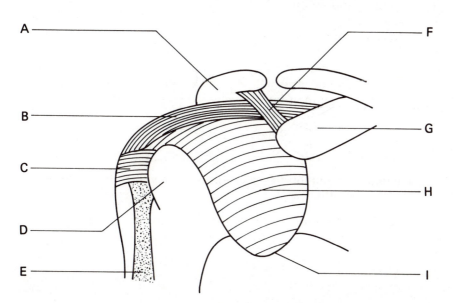

Fig. 7.2 *Frontal view of the shoulder joint*

A: acromion
B: coracohumeral ligament
C: transverse humeral
     ligament *(across bicipital groove)*
D: lesser tuberosity
E: long head of biceps

F: coracoacromial ligament
G: coracoid process
H: glenohumeral ligaments
I: joint capsule

THE ELBOW JOINTS

The elbow is a synovial joint consisting of two components: the humeroulnar joint is a hinge joint between the cylindrical trochlea of the humerus and the trochlear notch of the ulna; the humeroradial joint is a plane joint between the convex capitulum of the humerus and the flat head of the radius. The elbow joint allows flexion and extension of the forearm on the arm. The humeroradial joint and the proximal radioulnar joint together allow supination and pronation of the forearm.

The joint capsule is attached around the articular margins of the radius and ulna but has a more proximal attachment on the humerus which includes the radial, coronoid and olecranon fossae. Fat-pads separate the capsule from its synovial lining in these fossae (Fig. 7.3).

The radial collateral ligament is a thickening of the capsule lateral to the joint (Fig. 7.4). It is triangular, with its apex attached to the lateral epicondyle and its base to the annular ligament of the proximal radioulnar joint. The ulnar collateral ligament is a capsular thickening consisting of three bands connecting the medial epicondyle and the olecranon and coronoid processes.

Relations:

anterior:	median nerve	
	brachial artery	
	radial artery	
	ulnar artery	in the cubital fossa
	common interosseous artery	
	biceps tendon	
posterior:	triceps	
medial:	common flexor origin of the forearm muscles	
	ulnar nerve	
lateral:	common extensor origin of the forearm muscles	

Vascular anatomy:

arterial:	brachial artery
	radial artery
	ulnar artery
	profunda brachii artery
venous:	venae comitantes, corresponding to arteries
lymph:	axillary nodes

Methods of imaging the elbow joint: as for the shoulder joint, p.180

THE RADIOULNAR JOINTS

The radioulnar joints are synovial pivot joints between the radius and the ulna. The proximal joint is an articulation between the radial head, the radial notch of the ulna and the annular ligament. The distal joint is an articulation between the head of the ulna, the ulnar notch of the radius and the fibrocartilaginous articular disc which separates the head of the ulna from the radiocarpal joint. Together the joints allow supination and pronation of the forearm.

The proximal joint capsule consists of the annular ligament, which narrows distally to restrain the radial head. The annular ligament is attached to the anterior and posterior margins of the radial notch of the ulna and to the radial collateral ligament of the elbow joint. *Contiguous with elbow joint*

The fibrocartilaginous articular disc of the distal radioulnar joint is triangular, with its base attached to the medial surface of the distal radius and its apex to the ulnar styloid process. It completely separates the joint from the radiocarpal joint. The joint capsule is attached to the margins of the articular surfaces and to the periphery of the disc.

The interosseous membrane of the forearm is an accessory ligament for both joints.

Vascular anatomy: as for the elbow joint, opposite, and wrist joint, p.186

Methods of imaging the radioulnar joint: as for the shoulder joint, p.180

THE JOINTS OF THE WRIST

The wrist is a complex arrangement of synovial joints consisting of four components (Fig. 7.5): the radiocarpal joint is an ellipsoid joint between the concavity of the distal radius and the proximal row of carpal bones; the intercarpal joints are plane joints between the carpal bones; the carpometacarpal joints of the second to fifth metacarpals are plane joints between the distal row of carpal bones and the bases of the metacarpals; the intermetacarpal joints are plane joints between the bases of the second to fifth metacarpals. Together the joints allow flexion, extension, adduction, abduction and circumduction of the hand on the forearm.

The joint capsule of the radiocarpal joint is attached to the articular margins of the radius and the carpal bones, to the ulnar styloid process and to the periphery of the fibrocartilaginous disc of the distal radioulnar joint. It forms a recess between the ulnar styloid process and the triquetral bone which is filled by a fibrocartilaginous menis-

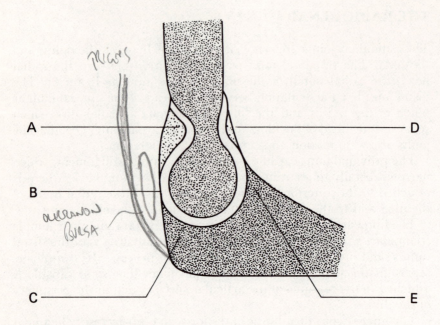

Fig. 7.3 *Parasagittal section through the humeroulnar joint*

A: posterior fat-pad in the
      olecranon fossa
B: joint capsule
C: olecranon process of the
      ulna

D: anterior fat-pad in the
      coronoid fossa
E: coronoid process of the
      ulna

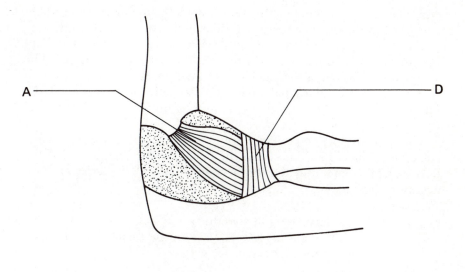

A ───────

D ───────

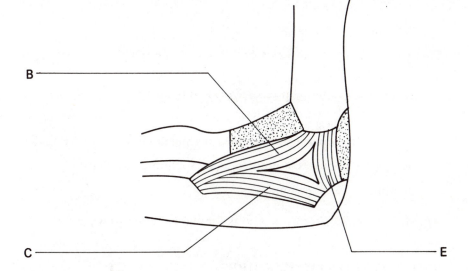

Fig. 7.4 *The elbow joint*

A: radial collateral ligament
B: anterior band of the ulnar
   collateral ligament
C: oblique band of the ulnar
   collateral ligament

D: annular ligament
E: posterior band of the
   ulnar collateral
   ligament

cus. The anterior and posterior radiocarpal ligaments and the radial and ulnar collateral ligaments are thickenings of the joint capsule.

The joint capsules of the intercarpal, carpometacarpal and intermetacarpal joints are attached to the articular margins. The synovial membrane of the carpometacarpal joints is continuous with that of the intermetacarpal joints and sometimes with that of the intercarpal joints. The dorsal and palmar ligaments are thickenings of the joint capsules.

The interosseous ligaments are numerous accessory ligaments connecting the carpal bones and the metacarpals. The tendon of the flexor carpi ulnaris and the flexor retinaculum of the wrist are also accessory ligaments.

Relations:

anterior: flexor tendon sheaths ⎫
median nerve   ⎬ in the carpal tunnel
*radial artery   ⎭

posterior: extensor muscles and tendons
abductor muscles and tendons
*radial artery

lateral: *radial artery

*The radial artery has a tortuous course around the wrist (see below).

Vascular anatomy:

arterial: anterior interosseous artery
radial artery
ulnar artery
superficial and deep palmer arches

venous: venae comitantes, corresponding to arteries

lymph: axillary nodes

Methods of imaging the wrist joints: as for the shoulder joint, p.180

THE ARTERIES OF THE UPPER LIMB

The axillary artery (Fig. 7.6) is the continuation of the subclavian artery beyond the outer border of the first rib. It traverses the axilla with the brachial plexus and axillary vein and gives branches to the thoracic wall, axillary structures and the shoulder joint.

The brachial artery is the continuation of the axillary artery beyond the lower border of the teres major. In the arm it is superficial and lies medial to the biceps muscle, with the median nerve. Its main branch is the profunda brachii artery which runs a spiral course in the radial groove of the humerus, with the radial nerve. The brachial artery divides into the radial and ulnar arteries in the cubital fossa.

The radial artery runs in the flexor compartment of the forearm, alongside the radial nerve, which is lateral to it. At the wrist it turns laterally around the radiocarpal joint on to the dorsum of the hand, then forward between the first and second metacarpals to enter the palm of the hand, where it ends as the deep palmar arch.

The ulnar artery also runs in the flexor compartment of the forearm, with the ulnar nerve on its medial side. Its main branch is the common interosseous artery, which arises in the cubital fossa and divides into anterior and posterior interosseous arteries. The ulnar artery enters the palm to the flexor retinaculum and divides into the superficial and deep palmar arches which anastomose with terminal branches of the radial artery.

Methods of imaging the arteries of the upper limb:

radiographic: arteriography

ultrasonographic: real-time B-mode
                     Doppler

THE VEINS OF THE UPPER LIMB

Most of the venous drainage of the upper limb is via a superficial network of veins which unite to form the basilic and cephalic veins (Fig. 7.7). The axillary vein is the continuation of the basilic vein above the lower border of the teres major muscle. The cephalic vein pierces the clavipectoral fascia before joining the axillary vein in the axilla.

Some venous drainage occurs via deep veins accompanying the arteries.

Methods of imaging the veins of the upper limb:

radiographic: ascending venography

ultrasonographic: real-time B-mode

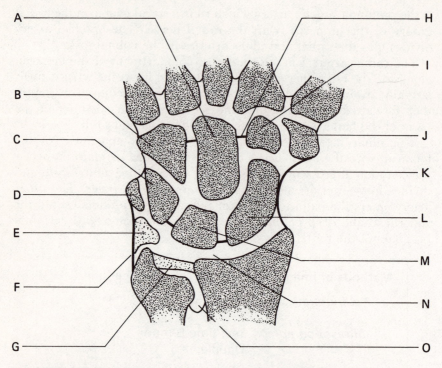

Fig. 7.5 *Coronal section through the wrist joints*

A: capitate
B: hamate
C: triquetral
D: pisiform
E: meniscus
F: ulnar collateral ligament
G: articular disc

H: interosseous ligament
I: trapezoid
J: trapezium
K: radial collateral ligament
L: scaphoid
M: lunate
N: radiocarpal joint
O: distal radioulnar joint

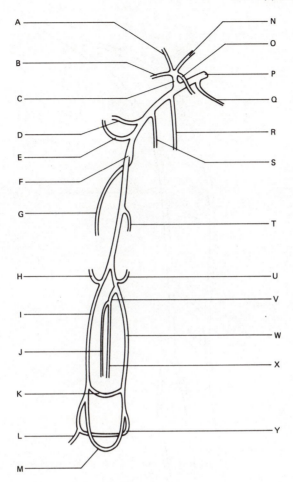

Fig. 7.6   *Arteries of the upper limb*

A: acromial artery
B: deltoid artery
C: acromiothoracic artery
D: posterior circumflex
      humeral artery
E: anterior circumflex
      humeral artery
F: brachial artery
G: profunda brachii artery
H: radial recurrent artery
I: radial artery
J: posterior interosseous
      artery
K: carpal arch
L: arteria princeps pollicis
M: superficial palmar arch

N: clavicular artery
O: pectoral artery
P: axillary artery
Q: superior thoracic artery
R: lateral thoracic artery
S: subscapular artery
T: ulnar collateral artery
U: ulnar recurrent artery
V: common interosseous
      artery
W: ulnar artery
X: anterior interosseous
      artery
Y: deep palmar arch

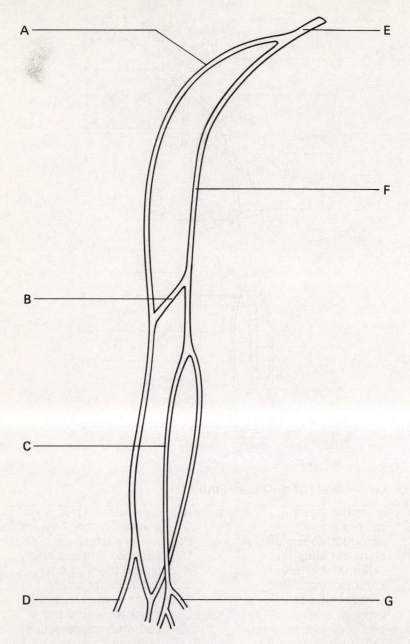

Fig. 7.7 *Veins of the upper limb*

A: cephalic vein
B: median cubital vein
C: median vein of the
        forearm
D: dorsal network

E: axillary vein
F: basilic vein
G: palmar plexus

8 | The Lower Limb

The lower limb supports the body in an upright position and is used for locomotion. The joints are stable and the muscles are powerful and fatigue-resistant. The fibres of the joint capsules and accessory ligaments are orientated so that they provide passive support when the body is erect but stationary.

THE HIP JOINTS

The hip joint is a synovial ball-and-socket joint between the concave acetabular fossa of the pelvic skeleton and the spherical head of the femur (Fig. 3.1). Despite having the stability required for weight-bearing it accommodates a wide range of movement.

The joint capsule is attached to the margin of the acetabular fossa and around the neck of the femur, extending as far as the inter-trochanteric line anteriorly. The retinacula are capsular fibres which extend from the margin of the capsule on the femoral neck into the joint, carrying blood vessels to the femoral head. The fibrocartila-ginous acetabular labrum is attached to the rim of the acetabular fossa, increasing the area of the articular surfaces and enveloping the head of the femur (Fig. 8.1). The ligament of the femoral head is a strong band connecting the femoral head to a notch in the acetatabu-lum. The synovial membrane of the joint forms a tubular sheath around the ligament.

The iliofemoral ligament is a triangular thickening of the joint capsule anteriorly, with its apex attached to the anterior superior iliac spine and its base attached to the upper femur between the greater and lesser trochanters (Fig. 8.2). The pubofemoral and ischiofemoral ligaments are inferior and posterior thickenings, respectively, of the joint capsule.

The ligament of the femoral head is the only accessory ligament.

Relations (Fig. 3.3):

  anterior: iliopsoas and pectineus
              femoral vein
              femoral artery   } *within femoral sheath*
              femoral nerve

  posterior: piriformis, obturator internus and quadratus femoris
              sciatic nerve
              gluteal muscles

Vascular anatomy:

  arterial: obturator artery
              superior gluteal artery
              inferior gluteal artery
              profunda femoris artery

  venous: venae comitantes, corresponding to arteries

  lymph: deep inguinal nodes
              internal iliac nodes

Methods of imaging the hip joint:

  radiographic: plain films and tomography
                    computed tomography
                    arthrography

  ultrasonographic: real-time B-mode in the
                        newborn

  radionuclide: ^{99m}Tc-diphosphonate bone
                    scintigraphy

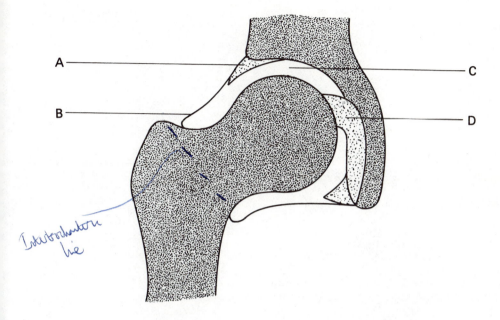

Fig. 8.1 *Coronal section through the hip joint*

A: acetabular labrum
B: joint capsule

C: acetabular fossa
D: ligament of the head of
    the femur

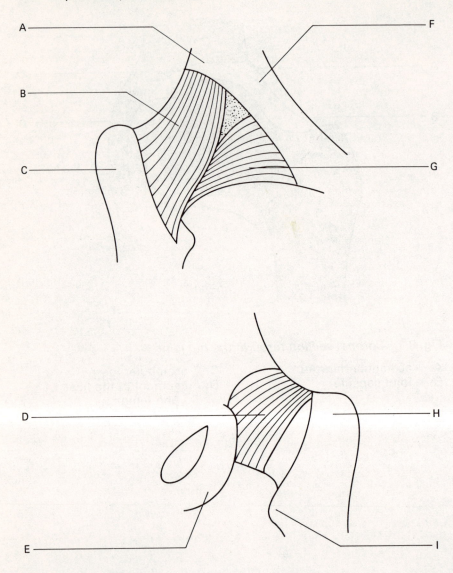

Fig. 8.2 *The hip joint*

A: anterior inferior iliac
        spine
B: iliofemoral ligament
C: greater trochanter
D: ischiofemoral ligament
E: ischial tuberosity

F: pubic ramus
G: pubofemoral ligament
H: greater trochanter
I: lesser trochanter

THE KNEE JOINTS

The knee joint is a synovial joint consisting of two condylar femoro-tibial components and a saddle-shaped patellofemoral component. The convex articular surfaces of the femoral condyles are continuous superiorly with the concave articular surface of the patellofemoral joint and are separated inferiorly and posteriorly by the intercondylar notch. The knee joint allows flexion of the leg on the thigh. Hyperextension of the knee is accompanied by external rotation of the tibia and 'locks' the knee, contributing to its stability on weight-bearing.

The joint capsule is attached to the articular margin and to the posterior limit of the intercondylar notch of the femur. It is attached to the articular margins of the patella and the tibial plateau, extending distally to include the tibial tuberosity. The menisci (Figs. 8.3, 8.5) are fibrocartilaginous crescents between the articular surfaces of the tibia and the femoral condyles. They are triangular in coronal section and the medial meniscus has a greater diameter than the lateral in transverse section. Each meniscus has an anterior and a posterior horn attached to the intercondylar area of the tibia and a rim attached to the tibial plateau by a coronary ligament. The anterior and posterior cruciate ligaments are attached to the intercondylar area of the tibia and to the femoral condyles. The anterior cruciate ligament resists anterior movement of the tibia on the femur and is attached to the lateral femoral condyle. The tendon of the popliteus muscle pierces the capsule posterolaterally and is attached to the lateral meniscus. Synovial membrane lines the joint except over the articular surfaces and menisci and has a complex arrangement (Figs. 8.3, 8.4): the suprapatellar bursa is a synovial recess above the patellofemoral component; the infrapatellar fold is a longitudinal fold of synovial membrane separating the tibiofemoral components of the joint, with the space between the components filled by a fat-pad and the cruciate ligaments.

The patellar ligament is an anterior thickening of the joint capsule attached to the apex of the patella and to the tibial tuberosity. The medial and lateral patellar retinacula are thickenings of the joint capsule on either side of the patellar ligament into which the vasti muscles are inserted. The tibial collateral ligament is a medial thickening of the capsule and the oblique popliteal ligament is a posterior thickening.

The fibular collateral ligament is an accessory ligament attached to the lateral femoral condyle and to the head of the fibula. The cruciate ligaments, coronary ligaments and menisci are also accessory ligaments.

Relations:

anterior: quadriceps muscles
            subcutaneous prepatellar bursa

posterior: popliteal artery ⎫
            popliteal vein   ⎬ in the popliteal fossa
            tibial nerve   ⎪
            lymph nodes   ⎭

Vascular anatomy:

arterial: profunda femoris artery
            genicular arteries
            anterior tibial recurrent artery

venous: venae comitantes, corresponding to arteries

lymph: popliteal node
            deep inguinal nodes

Methods of imaging the knee joint:

radiographic: plain films and tomography
                  computed tomography
                  arthrography

radionuclide: ^{99m}Tc-diphosphonate bone
                  scintigraphy

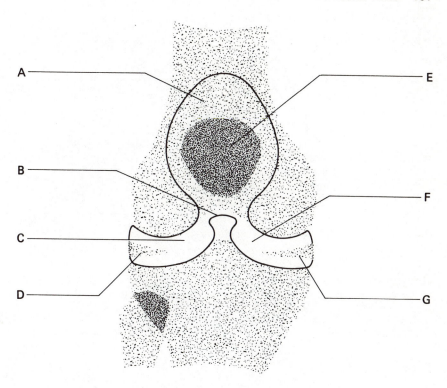

Fig. 8.3 *The arrangement of the synovial membrane of the knee*

A: suprapatellar bursa
B: infrapatellar fold
C: lateral joint compartment
D: lateral meniscus

E: patella
F: medial joint compartment
G: medial meniscus

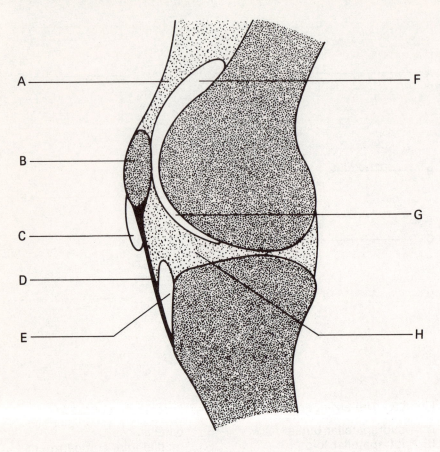

Fig. 8.4   *Parasagittal section through the knee joint*

A: quadriceps tendon
B: patella
C: subcutaneous prepatellar
       bursa
D: patellar ligament
E: deep infrapatellar bursa

F: suprapatellar bursa
G: infrapatellar fold
H: infrapatellar fat-pad

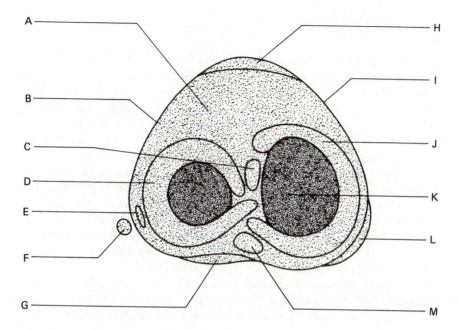

Fig. 8.5 *Cross section through the knee joint*

A: infrapatellar fat-pad
B: lateral patellar
       retinaculum
C: anterior cruciate ligament
D: lateral meniscus
E: popliteus tendon
F: fibular collateral ligament
G: oblique popliteal ligament

H: patellar ligament
I: medial patellar
       retinaculum
J: medial meniscus
K: femoral condyle
L: tibial collateral ligament
M: posterior cruciate
       ligament

THE ANKLE JOINTS

The ankle joint is a synovial hinge joint between the tibia, the fibula and the talus. The inferior surface of the tibia and the deep surfaces of the malleoli form a mortise above and on either side of the talus. The joint allows plantar flexion and dorsiflexion of the foot. The talus is broader anteriorly than posteriorly so that dorsiflexion is accompanied by 'locking' of the ankle joint, contributing to its stability on weight-bearing.

The joint capsule is attached to the articular margins and extends distally to the neck of the talus. The medial ligament is a triangular thickening of the capsule with its apex attached to the medial malleolus and its base to the sustentaculum tali of the calcaneus, the tuberosity of the navicular bone and the calcaneonavicular ligament (Fig. 8.6). The lateral ligament consists of three thickenings of the joint capsule arising from the fibula and attached to the anterior talus, the posterior talus and the calcaneus. The anterior and posterior ligaments are weak capsular thickenings.

The anterior, posterior and interosseous tibiofibular ligaments are accessory ligaments in front of, behind and above the joint, respectively. The inferior transverse tibiofibular ligament connects the malleoli, forming part of the posterior articular surface of the mortise.

Vascular anatomy:

arterial:	anterior tibial artery
	posterior tibial artery
	peroneal artery
venous:	venae comitantes, corresponding to arteries
lymph:	deep inguinal nodes

Methods of imaging the ankle joint: as for the knee joint, p.196

THE ARTERIES OF THE LOWER LIMB

The femoral artery (Fig. 8.7) is the continuation of the external iliac artery below the inguinal ligament. In the upper thigh it is superficial and lies between the femoral vein medially and the femoral nerve laterally. Its main branch is the profunda femoris artery. The femoral artery pierces the adductor magnus muscle 10 cm above the knee joint to enter the popliteal fossa.

The popliteal artery is the continuation of the femoral artery beyond the adductor magnus muscle. It traverses the popliteal fossa deep to the popliteal vein and divides into the anterior and posterior tibial arteries, its terminal branches.

The anterior tibial artery turns forward above the interosseous membrane and descends through the extensor compartment of the leg. It continues, as the dorsalis pedis artery, over the tarsal bones and enters the sole of the foot between the first and second metatarsals.

The posterior tibial artery descends in the flexor compartment of the leg to the medial malleolus. Its main branch is the peroneal artery, which descends behind the interosseous ligament. The posterior tibial artery divides into medial and lateral plantar arteries which anastomose with the dorsalis pedis artery.

Methods of imaging the arteries of the lower limb:

radiographic: femoral arteriography
                  translumbar aortography

ultrasonographic: real-time B-mode
                      Doppler

THE VEINS OF THE LOWER LIMB

Most of the venous drainage of the lower limb is via deep veins which accompany the correspondingly-named arteries and which drain venous plexuses related to the muscles of the calf and thigh (Fig. 8.8).

The superficial venous drainage consists of the long and short saphenous veins draining into the femoral and popliteal veins, respectively. The superficial and deep veins also communicate via perforating vessels, whose valves allow blood to flow from the superficial to the deep system.

Methods of imaging the veins of the lower limb:

radiographic: ascending and descending
                  venography

ultrasonographic: real-time B-mode

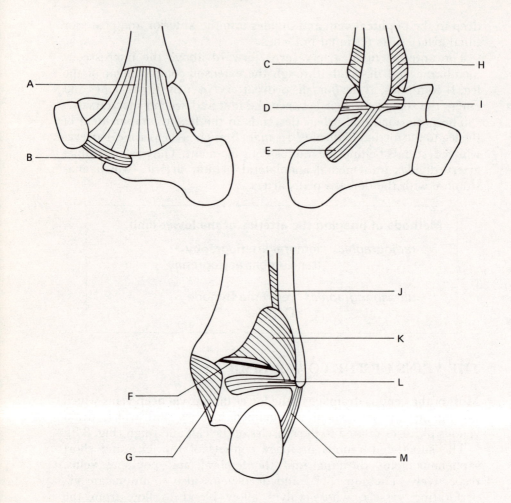

Fig. 8.6   *The ankle joint*

A: medial ligament
B: plantar calcaneonavicular
      ligament
C: posterior tibiofibular
      ligament
D: posterior talofibular
      ligament (lateral
      ligament)
E: calcaneofibular ligament
      (lateral ligament)
F: inferior transverse
      ligament
G: medial ligament

H: anterior tibiofibular
      ligament
I: anterior talofibular
      ligament (lateral
      ligament)
J: interosseous ligament/
      membrane
K: posterior tibiofibular
      ligament
L: posterior talofibular
      ligament
M: calcaneofibular ligament

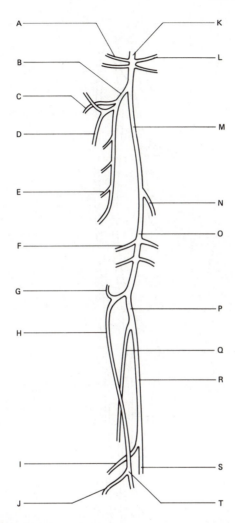

Fig. 8.7   *Arteries of the lower limb*

A: circumflex iliac arteries
B: profunda femoris artery
C: medial circumflex femoral
    artery
D: lateral circumflex femoral
    artery
E: perforating branches
F: genicular arteries
G: anterior tibial recurrent
    artery
H: anterior tibial artery
I: lateral plantar arch
J: arcuate artery

K: femoral artery
L: external pudendal arteries
M: superficial femoral artery
N: descending genicular
    artery
O: popliteal artery
P: common peroneal artery
Q: peroneal artery
R: posterior tibial artery
S: medial plantar artery
T: dorsalis pedis artery

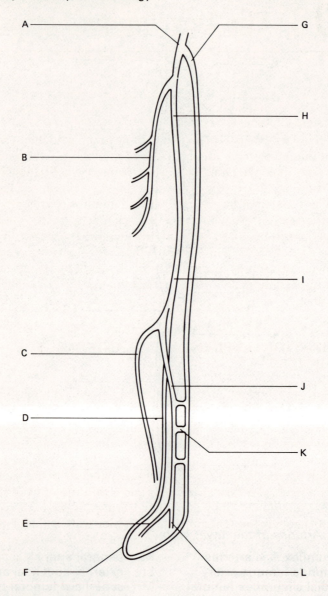

Fig. 8.8 *Veins of the lower limb*

A: common femoral vein
B: profunda femoris vein
C: anterior tibial vein
D: short saphenous vein
E: lateral plantar vein
F: dorsal venous arch

G: long saphenous vein
H: superficial femoral vein
I: popliteal vein
J: posterior tibial vein
K: perforating vein
L: medial plantar vein

9 | The Developing Fetus

The product of fertilization of an ovum by a spermatozoon is a zygote, a single totipotential cell which develops into the mature fetus, its coverings and the placenta. In early pregnancy cell division and differentiation result in the formation of specialized tissues and organs. The conceptus has a recognizable human form eight weeks after fertilization and from this time is known as a fetus.

Ultrasonography is used to demonstrate the conceptus in early pregnancy and to image the anatomy of the fetus in later pregnancy. The following section is a brief account of the embryology of each system and a description of the fetal anatomy 14 weeks after fertilization.

FERTILIZATION, IMPLANTATION AND EARLY DEVELOPMENT

Fertilization of the ovum occurs in the lateral part of the uterine tube within 24 hours of ovulation. The single-celled conceptus undergoes several divisions, resulting in the formation of the morula, an amorphous mass of cells, which enters the uterine cavity three days after fertilization. Further cell division and the development of a cavity result in the formation of the blastocyst, an ovoid structure containing a mass of embryogenic cells and a thin rim of trophoblasts which subsequently develops into the coverings of the embryo (Fig. 9.1). The blastocyst implants into the posterior wall of the uterus six days after fertilization, whereupon the trophoblasts proliferate and fuse to form the multinucleated syncytiotrophoblast, which is bathed by maternal blood.

After implantation the embryogenic cells differentiate into ectoderm and endoderm and the amniotic cavity develops. With further growth and development the original cavity of the blastocyst is reorganized to form the yolk sac. Two weeks after fertilization the embryo consists of the germ disc, a double-layered structure of ectoderm and endoderm, which separates the amniotic cavity from the yolk sac. These structures are connected, by a stalk, to the covering of the embryo, now known as the chorion. Further growth causes elongation of the germ disc. Differentiation of the ectoderm results in the formation of the neural tube and the notochord which give rise to neuroectoderm and mesoderm, respectively. The meso-derm undergoes segmentation along the length of the embryo, each segment consisting of paired somites on either side of the notochord. The formation of the head and tail folds and the two lateral body folds encloses a 'U'-shaped cavity which will develop into the pericardium, pleurae and peritoneum. As folding progresses the amniotic cavity expands and the yolk sac becomes contained within the embryo and connecting stalk. Four weeks after fertilization the embryo is com-posed of the four germ layers from which all tissues develop and is connected to its coverings by the umbilical cord.

Subsequent development results in the formation of organs and systems.

THE CIRCULATORY SYSTEM

The heart, pericardium, blood vessels and erythropoietic and lympho-poietic tissues are derived from mesoderm. A rudimentary circulation is established within four weeks of fertilization.

The heart initially consists of a single tube which invaginates into the pericardium. Blood enters via two vessels at the caudal end and is expelled into two ventral aortae at the cranial end. The heart tube elongates and develops into a four-chambered structure by a process of folding and by the formation of septa and valves. Axial rotation of the folded tube results in the definitive position of the cardiac chambers, with each ventricle becoming anterior to the corresponding atrium.

Each ventral aorta is connected to the corresponding dorsal aorta by six aortic arches. These give rise to the pulmonary and systemic circuits. Venous return comprises blood from the umbilical cord, the yolk sac and the fetal tissues, conveyed in paired umbilical, vitelline and common cardinal veins, respectively. The right umbilical vein becomes obliterated and the vitelline veins develop into the portal venous system.

Eight weeks after fertilization the definitive fetal circulation has developed (Fig. 9.2). The fetus derives all the raw materials for growth and development from, and excretes all its waste products into, the maternal blood at the placental insertion. Enriched blood from the placenta passes via the umbilical vein, the ductus venosus and the inferior vena cava to the right atrium and is directed into the left atrium through the foramen ovale, a defect in the interatrial septum. From here it passes to the left ventricle and is distributed through the systemic circulation, with the larger proportion entering the great vessels of the neck to supply the rapidly-developing brain. Venous blood from the brain returns via the superior vena cava to the right atrium, where there is only minimal mixing with the enriched blood from the inferior vena cava. It enters the right ventricle and returns via the pulmonary artery, ductus arteriosus, descending aorta, iliac arteries and umbilical arteries to the placenta. Only a small proportion enters the lungs, via constricted pulmonary arterioles. At birth adult circulation is established by the closure of the ductus arteriosus and the foramen ovale, accompanied by expansion and perfusion of the lungs. Following clamping of the umbilical cord the ductus venosus closes and the umbilical arteries and vein become obliterated.

THE ALIMENTARY AND RESPIRATORY SYSTEMS

The pharyngeal part of the alimentary and respiratory tracts develops from arches of endoderm and mesoderm. The larynx develops as a ventral diverticulum of endoderm which grows caudally and bifurcates to produce the lung buds. The respiratory passages result from further branching of the endoderm of the lung buds and the lung parenchyma is derived from mesoderm.

The yolk sac becomes the foregut and the hindgut, whose junction is marked by the vitellointestinal duct, the remnant of the yolk sac in the umbilical cord. The alimentary tract becomes continuous with the amniotic cavity with the perforation of the oropharyngeal and cloacal membranes. The midgut develops between the foregut and the hindgut and as it elongates it herniates into the umbilical cord. This hernia exists between five and 12 weeks after fertilization and, on reduction, rotation occurs.

The biliary system develops from a ventral diverticulum of foregut endoderm and the liver parenchyma is derived from mesoderm.

THE UROGENITAL SYSTEM

The mesoderm of the abdominal cavity gives rise to the pronephros, mesonephros and metanephros, successively. The definitive kidney and ureter develop from the metanephros and additional mesoderm. The epithelium of the bladder, prostate and most of the urethra is derived from the endoderm of the cloaca, with a small contribution of mesoderm forming the trigone of the bladder.

The epididymis, vas deferens, ejaculatory duct and seminal vesicle develop from the mesonephros, which forms a vestigial structure in the female. The testis develops from the mesoderm of the abdominal cavity and is attached to the anterior abdominal wall by the gubernaculum. The testis descends as far as the deep inguinal ring in the 24 weeks following fertilization, after which rapid descent into the scrotum occurs.

Paramesonephric ducts develop, in the female, from mesoderm of the abdominal cavity. The caudal parts of these ducts fuse to form the uterus and an ingrowth of ectoderm develops into the vagina. The ovary, like the testis, is derived from mesoderm of the abdominal cavity but descends only as far as the pelvis.

The male and female external genitalia follow parallel developmental pathways until eight weeks after fertilization, when they differentiate under the influence of sex hormones.

THE NERVOUS SYSTEM

The nervous system is derived from neuroectoderm, which forms the neural tube. The ends of the neural tube close within four weeks of fertilization and three swellings develop at its cranial end which give rise to the forebrain, midbrain and hindbrain. The cerebral hemispheres, the diencephalon and the third and lateral ventricles are derived from the forebrain. The cerebellum and its peduncles, the pons, medulla oblongata and the fourth ventricle are derived from the hindbrain. Growth of these structures is accompanied by folding of the tube and the disproportionate increase in surface area of the cerebral cortex is accommodated by the formation of sulci and gyri, commencing with the lateral sulcus 12 weeks after fertilization.

The retina and optic nerve develop from diverticula of the forebrain. The lens and cornea are derived from ectoderm and the uveal tract from mesoderm.

The dura mater and the choroid plexus are derived from mesoderm and the arachnoid mater and pia mater from neuroectoderm.

THE MUSCULOSKELETAL SYSTEM

Muscle, bone, cartilage, synovium and connective tissue are all derived from mesoderm and are organized on a segmental basis. The limb buds begin to develop within four weeks of fertilization and the definitive limbs are recognizable eight weeks after fertilization. Ossification of each long bone begins at the primary centre, in the shaft, and is followed by ossification of the epiphyses. The first primary ossification centre to develop is that of the clavicle, six weeks after fertilization. Ossification of the distal femoral and proximal tibial epiphyses occurs shortly before term.

THE UMBILICAL CORD AND PLACENTA

The chorion forms the outer covering of the fetus and is derived from trophoblastic cells and mesodermal cells. The chorion in the region of the connecting stalk develops villi which are bathed by maternal blood. As the amniotic cavity expands the chorion becomes lined by the amnion, a membrane derived from ectodermal cells, which extends to cover the placenta and umbilical cord.

The placenta is connected to the fetus by the umbilical cord, which consists of two umbilical arteries, a single left umbilical vein and the vitellointestinal duct, supported within the amnion by Wharton's jelly. The right umbilical vein is obliterated. At term the umbilical cord is 50 cm long and the placenta is 20 cm in diameter.

THE FETUS IN THE EARLY SECOND TRIMESTER

Fourteen weeks after fertilization (16 weeks after the last menstrual period) all the definitive structures and organs have developed and fetal anatomy differs from that of the adult mainly in bodily proportions. If the fetus is imaged it is possible to demonstrate fetal activity, the beating heart, respiratory activity and swallowing.

The heart occupies a large proportion of the thorax since the lungs are not aerated. As a consequence of placental circulation the right and left ventricular walls are of similar thickness and the ductus arteriosus is patent.

The abdominal circumference is less than that of the head owing to the preferential growth of the nervous system. As pregnancy progresses, however, abdominal growth accelerates, mainly because of expansion of the liver, which occupies a large proportion of the abdomen (Fig. 9.3). The umbilical vein passes upward and backward through the liver to join the left branch of the portal vein, which is connected to the inferior vena cava by the ductus venosus. Paired umbilical arteries, branches of the internal iliac arteries, pass lateral to the bladder to enter the umbilical cord. The kidneys are lobulated and the adrenal glands are proportionally larger than in the adult. The external genitalia are sufficiently developed for the sex of the fetus to be determined, though the testes are still intra-abdominal.

In the fetal brain the septum pellucidum consists of two layers separated by the cavum septi pellucidi, a narrow, fluid-filled cavity in the midline. Expansion of the cerebral cortex has produced the lateral sulcus and the insula but other sulci and gyri are not yet present. As growth proceeds the ventricular system occupies a diminishing proportion of brain volume: each lateral ventricle should extend from the midline to occupy 60% of the width of each hemisphere.

The limbs are fully developed but the upper limbs are larger than the lower. Primary ossification of several long bones is well advanced and allows the length of the femur to be used as a measure of maturity. The facial structures are fully developed, though the eyes are more widely spaced than in the adult.

The placenta lies in a variable position on the posterior wall of the uterus, extending down from the fundus occasionally as far as the internal os. The volume of amniotic fluid depends, in part, on the integrity of the alimentary and renal tracts.

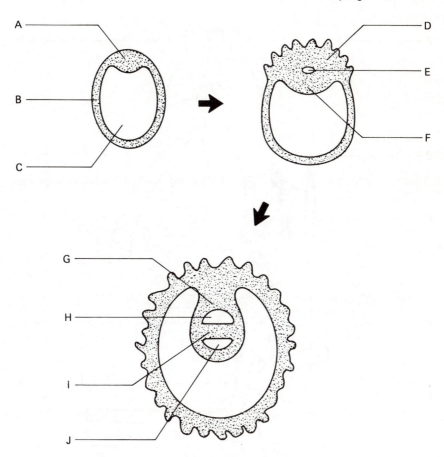

Fig. 9.1 *Development of the blastocyst*

A: embryogenic cells
B: trophoblasts
C: cavity of the blastocyst
D: syncytiotrophoblast
E: amniotic cavity

F: germ disc
G: connecting stalk
H: amniotic cavity
I: germ disc
J: yolk sac

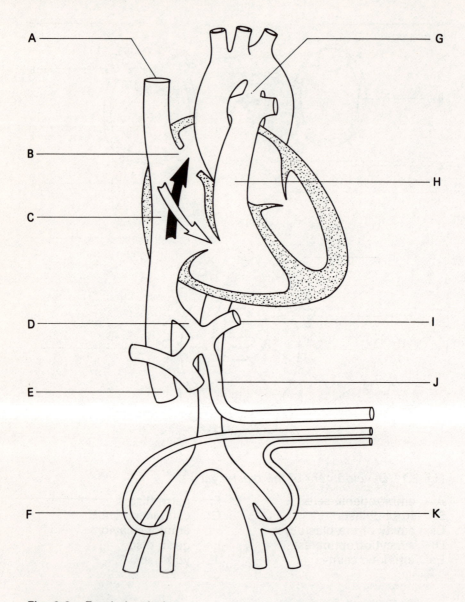

Fig. 9.2 *Fetal circulation*

A: superior vena cava
B: foramen ovale
C: right atrium
D: ductus venosus
E: inferior vena cava
F: right umbilical artery

G: ductus arteriosus
H: pulmonary artery
I: left branch of the portal
    vein
J: umbilical vein
K: left umbilical artery

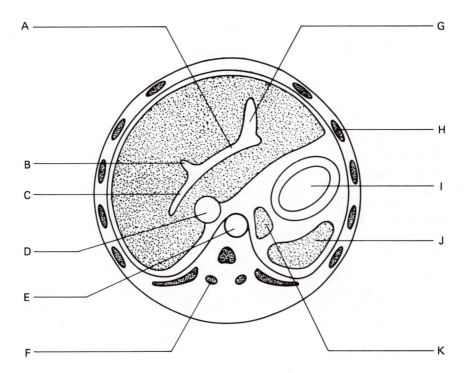

Fig. 9.3   *Cross section through the fetal abdomen*

A: left branch of the portal
      vein
B: anterior branch of the
      right portal vein
C: posterior branch of the
      right portal vein
D: inferior vena cava
E: aorta
F: primary vertebral
      ossification centre

G: umbilical vein
H: rib
I: stomach
J: spleen
K: left adrenal gland

Index